I'm a Teen! Now What?
A Survival Guide for Teenage Girls

Foreword by

Juliette Brindak
Star of BBC's Million Dollar Intern &
CEO & Co-Founder of 'Miss O & Friends'

Greg & Cristina Noland

www.OMGTeenBookSeries.com

OMG – I'm A Teen! – Now What?
A Survival Guide for Teenage Girls

Authors: Greg & Cristina Noland
Foreword by Juliette Brindak

Second Edition
ISBN-13:
978-1511442985
ISBN-10:
1511442980

Published by **Red Scorpion Marketing & Publishing Ltd**
info@redscorpionmarketing.com
22 Bentinck Lane, East Lane, Hull, East Riding of Yorkshire, HU11 5QR

Tel: +44 (0) 560 367 9116 / +66 (0) 09 008 7070

E-mails: greg@omgteenbookseries.com / cristina@omgteenbookseries.com
Web: www.omgteenbookseries.com

MEDICAL AND GENERAL DISCLAIMER FOR THE BUM GUN LTD

The Bum Gun Ltd is intended for informational purposes only. Our books and websites contain general information about health, hygiene, medical conditions and treatments, and provide information and ideas for, but not limited to, improving the quality of life for every individual.

The Bum Gun Ltd makes no claims that anything presented is true, accurate, proven, and/or not harmful to your health or wellbeing. Our books and websites are not and do not claim to be written, edited, or researched by a health care professional.

Any information on or associated with this website should NOT be considered a substitute for medical advice from a healthcare professional. If you are experiencing any form of health problem, always consult a doctor before attempting any treatment on your own. The Bum Gun Ltd will not be held liable or responsible in any way for any harm, injury, illness, or death that may result from the use of its content or anything related to it.

Viewers assume all risk and liability associated with the use of the content on our books and websites, and must agree to our terms and conditions.

DISCLAIMER ON COMMENTS & ADVICE GIVEN

Please note that the below information is designed to provide general information on the topics presented. It is provided with the understanding that the expert is not engaged in rendering any medical or professional services in the information provided below. The information provided should not be used as a substitute for professional services.

Table of Contents

Foreword

By Juliette Brindak

Star of BBC's Million Dollar Intern & CEO & Co-Founder of 'Miss O & Friends'

Hi everyone! My name is Juliette Brindak and I would like to introduce this first book in the OMG Teen Book Series: *"OMG I'm A Teen. Now What? - A Survival Guide For Female Teens."* I was first introduced to the author of this book, Greg Noland through my work on the hit British TV show *Million Dollar Intern.* Greg knew about my work helping tweens through my own website, Miss O & Friends® (www.MissO.com) and approached me to work on this book together.

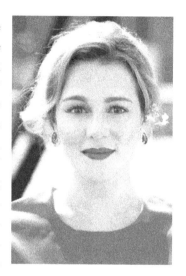

Middle school was tough times. I call it tough times because middle school sucks. Girls go through a lot during in these years. That awkward phase kicks in. Boys come into the picture. Cliques begin to form. School becomes more serious. Bullying increases. Girls start to struggle with self-esteem & the pressure to fit in. It doesn't matter if a girl is the most popular girl in school or the best athlete or a band geek or a straight-A student or a punk. No matter who she is doesn't make her any more, or less, vulnerable to feeling insecure. Inspired by my sister Olivia (the real Miss O) and her friends, Miss O & Friends® was started to create a safe place online for girls to *just* be girls. As we aim to help build self-esteem while still being fun, entertaining, and helpful destination for tween & teen girls, our goal is help girls get through this tough period of their lives a little happier, more secure and empowered. Greg's OMG Teen Book Series is the perfect complement to my own work and with the female perspective from his wife Cristina, it's perfect for tween & teen girls who are looking for more answers.

Obviously I was a teen with lots of issues and troubles to face just like you. Luckily I had a very supportive family to help guide me through all those troublesome teenage years. And now as a successful entrepreneur I know the importance of having the right knowledge at your fingertips. Through my work with Miss O & Friends®, and talking with so many tweens & teens, I know so many girls just don't have the vital information and support I was lucky to have.

I am so happy that Greg has worked so hard to put this book together and is so passionate about helping so many people as possible through his whole OMG Teen Book Series to help shed light on those questions teens are desperately seeking answers too!

I know how teen girls can face all sorts of issues like struggling with self-esteem, spells of depression, trouble with self-confidence, this book will help keep you going when you hit those brick walls, and propel to your real self.

"Take success and failures as they come, since things often change at a moment's notice."

xoxo,

Juliette

Introduction

Thank you and Congratulations for purchasing this book *'OMG – I'm A Teen! – Now What? A Survival Guide for Teenage Girls'*. This is not just any book; this is the book that will ultimately give you the tools to live a much fuller and more rewarding life.

This book represents nearly 20 years of hard work, experiences and the efforts of my network of friends, family, and colleagues and of course my incredible customers who I owe so much for believing in me. Maybe you're one of them!

How did this book and the 'OMG Teen Book Series' get started? You might be wondering... what gives me the authority to write this book? Well, in fact the credit for the initial start for this book goes to my best friend's daughter, Annabelle. As all teens realise, being a teen can be really tough. During a particular difficult period for Annabelle, it seemed like she was coming to me every few days for advice. Don't get me wrong, I loved that she trusted my advice and that I could help her. But I thought I could possibly help her more by guiding her to a book or two targeted at helping teens improve the quality of their lives. After searching the local book stores, libraries and then online, I could not find anything suitable at all. Suddenly, I remembered something Jack Canfield, the author of 'Chicken Soup for the Soul' once told me, and that was if you can't find the book, then you are destined to write it.

You might also be thinking it is strange for a guy to be writing a survival guide for teenage girls. Well, I had always intended writing some books, though not specifically on this subject area. I didn't really feel I had the complete authority to write a book aimed at female teenagers.

Consequently, I set about interviewing as many females in my family and network as I could, and the immense support I received from them gave me the confidence to get to writing. So a huge thank you to all female members of my family, friends and network. You all rock!

I would like to give an extra special thank you to Juliette Brindak for agreeing to work with me on this book. As a very successful entrepreneur, I understand how super busy Juliette is every day. So taking the time out to contribute to this book, and give her unique knowledge of helping teenagers has been supremely valuable. Thank you Juliette. Please check out her Miss O & Friends® website at www.MissO.com

And obviously a huge thanks needs to be reserved for my lovely wife Cristina who helped me with all the specific female areas of this book. You did an amazing job. The fantastic thing is that so many adult females who read the launch version of this book have said they learned so much from the natural beauty and make up tips in Chapter 4 so that's double fantastic. So I'm super stoked teens as well as adult can benefit from this book.

Life Is About Learning Through Access To Information

Hey! Welcome to the wonderful time of being a teen. You have entered a time in your life that is exciting and scary at the same time. New things start happening to your body, new things that are changing your life, new adventures to discover, and often a lot of new responsibilities. This is definitely an exciting but scary time for you.

Chances are that you have questions that you want to ask and things that you need to know about. This is why we have created this book; to help you understand and have your questions answered. We are going to cover things like hygiene, your period, makeup, responsibilities, and many other things that are going to give you the best chances to be successful during your teen years. We are also going to give you some advice on school and hopefully answer some of the questions that you have wanted to ask but have been afraid to up to now.

I understand there are some people who like to make their own mistakes in life and prefer to ignore the advice from others. Perhaps then, this book might not be for those of you who are of this mannerism.

But there is a large number of people who would rather listen, learn and push ahead with their lives using any rich knowledge they can find to increase their chances of success, improve the quality of their lives and decrease states of pain, sadness, mistakes and regrets. If you think you are in this group of successful go-getters, then this book is definitely for you.

Lessons From My Teen Years

I wouldn't say I had a totally unhappy childhood, because I guess many people have had much more pain and sadness than me. But it was indeed loaded with many problems, mistakes, and upsetting situations that I would never wish on anyone.

I know most children have issues and problems in their lives, and I guess dealing with these difficult situations is what moulds us into who we are as adults.

However, now that I am an adult, in hindsight I know that my childhood and particularly my teen years would have been much easier, much happier, and ultimately more successful if I had the right information to guide me along the right path.

Even though I came from a fairly big family, with many siblings, my family was just not the kind where you would ask for or share advice. I am not sure if it was the divorce of my parents when I was 8 years old, or due to being the youngest in the family, but I often felt lost, lonely, and confused.

I often felt that no one had the same feelings as me regarding growing up. I also felt there was no one there to help me with the problems of being a teenager, and what I wanted to do with my life. I think because of my parents' divorce I had to grow up so much quicker than other people, so it felt like everyone around me at school were so much younger than me. This further compounded the problem of loneliness and the shortage of helpful information. Of course, I didn't have the use of the Internet back then.

I know being brought up in a single parent family is much more common these days, but I very much doubt it is any easier. Being a lone parent is surely a very difficult task, and try as they might to be the dad, the mum, the child counsellor, the leader and the friend, there is bound to be big chunks missing from the life of a teenager from a single parent family. This is where this book can truly help fill in those gaps.

Who can you turn to when you are faced with traumatic experiences in your teenage years?

I can still remember to this day the people who bullied me. I can remember their exact names. I remember the rocks being thrown at me, and the pain of those rocks hitting my body. I remember like it was yesterday as a group ripped off my new school blazer and dragged it through a muddy puddle. I can still feel the thud of kicks hitting my body, one after the other. I can remember my school bag being slashed by a gang of older kids for no other reason than "they felt like it".

Whether you have been unfortunate enough to be a victim of bullying or have had other difficult issues, every adult has been where you are right now and we understand what you are going through. So sit back and please enjoy reading this book. We hope that you will find it very informative and that many of your questions will be answered. It is our mission to ensure that the information, advice and tips contained in this book will act as effective resources to help you through your teenage years, and makes you realise that you are not alone. The Survival Guide for Teenage Girls will give you the strength to overcome some of the difficult problems you may have to face as a teenager.

I am delighted the exceptional entrepreneur Juliette Brindak, Star of BBC's Million Dollar Intern & CEO & Co-Founder of 'Miss O & Friends' has agreed to work with us on this book. Please read her foreword in this book for more information.

Once again, thank you to my wonderful wife for helping me with all the specific female areas of this book.

Dedicated to your happy and successful life,

Greg Noland
Founder and CEO - The Bum Gun

Chapter 1
Why Has Life Suddenly Become So Difficult?

"People seem to forget that these lovely babies and toddlers grow up fast and can have a demon on their hands before they know it!!"
This is a common thought for many parents. Suddenly, the super sweet, cuddly cutie doesn't want to spend any time with their parents, and in some cases their child can become angry, aggressive and often speak very badly.

You might think you don't understand your parents right now, but in reality the person who is changing the most right now is you. Once you become a teen, your hormone balances change significantly, and so your moods can change rapidly for no apparent reason. Things which never used to bother you can suddenly become a big deal.

Your parents always want what is best for you. And now that you are a teenager, your whole life is opening up, and the opportunities open to you can be immense. This is why your parents are willing to put themselves out massively for you. Most teens suddenly have a huge variety of hobbies and outside of school activities they are interested in. Suddenly it seems you want to try everything, from learning musical instruments, ballet or dance classes, to cheerleading and martial arts.

The thing that hurts parents the most is that they work their behinds off to keep a roof over your head, bring you everything and I mean everything, make sure you can go pretty much everywhere you want, take you to nice places, help with your homework, and taxi you and your friends round. In return all they ask is that you respect them, and appreciate everything they do for you. It is absolute torture for a parent to have any kind of argument with their children whether you realise this right now, or not. So NEVER turn round and say you hate them or even worse wish they were dead, however angry and upset you may feel you are. Please try to be a little more easy-going and respectful should you ever disagree about anything with your parents.

Just remember that the whole world does not revolve only around you. Your parents have a life too and they cannot be expected to stop living it because they had you. More often than not, both your parents are working, and in the current world economy that probably means they are working harder than ever, and under more pressure and stress than at any other time in their lives.

Often during your teen years you will come across many kinds of new situations and problems, and your parents will try hard to show you that life is not about giving you everything on a plate and that you have to work for a better life. If they just gave you everything on a platter, they would not be preparing you well for your future. This will be difficult to understand right now, but please remember this chapter when you come up against this kind of situation with your parents.

Why Is My Relationship With My Mum So Hard?

One of the biggest difficulties with being a teenager is finding the right crowd to hang with. In my own experience, and from what my research shows, most people feel they made some terrible choices about friends when they were teenagers. It's really important to a teenager to be able to choose their own friends. However, it is really easy to fall in with the wrong crowd.

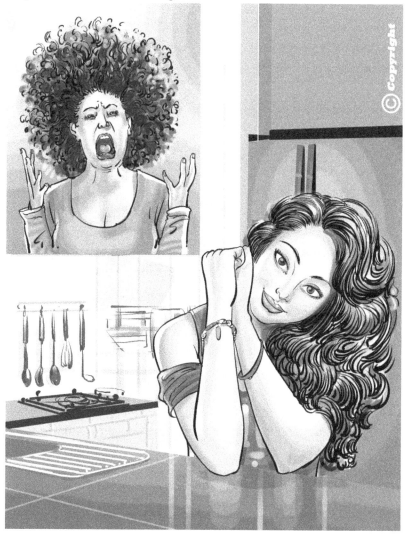

This could lead to numerous bad situations, because you might think you believe in your new "friends". But it is very hard to see how these situations can turn out. Later, you'll often wish you didn't waste so much time with these so-called friends and that you could have broken away from them sooner. So, next time you have a 'conversation' with your parents because they might not be happy with your new friends, listen to them. Do not get angry. Listen to the reasons as to why they think you should be careful about these friends. Remember, your parents have been through all these problems before, so they really DO have the experience to help guide you through these difficult choices. And yes, it is difficult to say no to your peers, and requires you to be really strong and mature.

Some Other Possible Disagreements With Your Parents

Piercings: Ouch That's Gotta Hurt

- Whether ears or navel (belly) piercings, they will hurt, after all you are putting a very sharp needle through your skin. Don't feel bad if your parents don't want you to get your belly pierced.
- Belly piercings take a deceptively long time to heal.
- Don't think about having a piercing right before a holiday. It's recommended to get it done at least 6 weeks before you go on holiday because the seawater/chlorine can mess it up, and there's bacteria in there which you don't want to get into a brand new piercing.

- Yes, belly piercings often go gammy, and will probably scar.
- Guys might think they look cheap as they are nothing new.

Tattoos: Yes, They're Forever!

I would recommend waiting at least 30 days if right now you think you want a tattoo, and a certain design. Your feelings will change about getting a tattoo full-stop, and especially the design. Getting a tattoo or not is one of those decisions in life which can come back to bite you if you are not very careful. If I had a dollar for every person who later regretted getting a tattoo I'd be very rich.

However small, you'll most likely regret your decision. My advice would be: Resist the urge.

Alcohol: How It Affects Your Body

According to the Archives of Paediatrics and Adolescent Medicine, almost 80% of teenagers have experimented with alcohol by the time they are 16. Even more disturbing are the statistics regarding accidents, violence and self-inflicted injuries among teenagers who abuse alcohol. Alcohol plays a role in more than 30 percent of teen-age deaths involving accidents, homicide or suicide.

Many teenagers do not realize that alcohol can interfere with their body's development. Drinking can cause weight gain, which may put you at risk for developing high blood pressure and type 2 diabetes. If teenagers keep drinking into adulthood they have a higher risk of developing cirrhosis of the liver when they're older. The liver is one of the most important organs in your body, helping you metabolize nutrients and rid your system of harmful toxins.

Alcohol can also kill your brain cells. Recent neurological research indicates that teenagers may be more prone to alcohol-related neurological damage than adults. A teenager's brain is at a vulnerable stage of development and alcohol interferes with this development, causing permanent changes in the ability to learn and remember.

- Resist the urge as drinking when you are young can do irreversible damage to your body.
- Resist the urge; all drugs are dangerous and will ruin your life quicker than you can imagine.

I believe being a teenager can be a very turbulent stage in most people's lives, but I know one thing and that is that life does improve a lot after your teen years. That was definitely the case for me. So if you feel life is unbearably hard right now, hang in there, it will improve very soon.

You will often find later in life that popularity is not all it's cracked up to be. As long as you feel happy with yourself and your friends, it doesn't matter how popular you are. The key is finding a group of people you can feel at ease being yourself with.

Chapter 2
Why Is Your Body Changing So Much?

As a teenager your body is going through a lot of changes to prepare you to become an adult with the ability of having a baby. This chapter is all about some of the changes going on with your body right now, starting with an interesting cause and effect situation related to toilet paper use.

Why Do Female Teens Use So Much Toilet Paper?

A little known fact is that female teens are by far the biggest users of toilet paper. Research says female teens can easily go through go through a roll of toilet paper about 6-8 times faster than a male teen. I have had customers tell me that one female teen in their house can go through as much as 1 or 2 rolls per day at some times during the month. With two female teens and mum in the house, then you could easily be going through a Costco bale of toilet paper a week. When I found these facts out, I promised myself to do a lot more research on this topic as this 'excessive' use is clearly a message that female teens have different personal hygiene needs to most guys. And improving people's personal hygiene is my business!!

So Where Does All That Toilet Paper Go?

For a start, females use way more toilet paper than men, pretty much as a rule, because of anatomy and also because of menstruation. Perhaps the biggest reason though for the high rate of usage among female teens is that there is so much change going on in your body.

You might be feeling yucky when you are having your periods and you are desperate to feel fresh between tampon or pad changes. Obviously it is not always easy to have a shower during the day, which is one of the main reasons the bidet sprayer was invented.

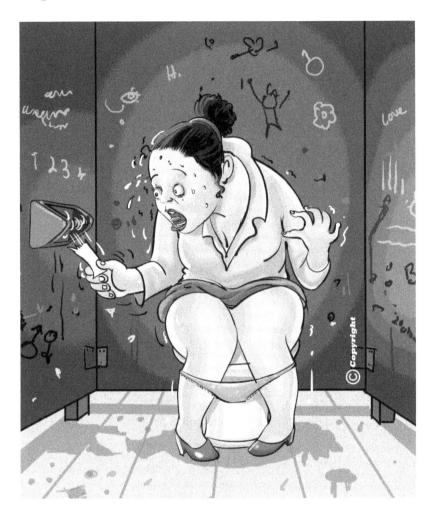

With this clever device, you can clean front and back while you are sat on the toilet and practically still fully clothed.

It is completely natural to want to feel "shower fresh" clean throughout the day. Having lived in Thailand for a lot of my life where the bidet sprayer is present in almost every bathroom, I still find it very strange that the western countries have still not caught up with this invention yet.

Most people only use a thickness of a few sheets to wipe themselves after the toilet. But research tells us that the germs in faeces come through as many as 10 sheets of toilet paper, so correct hand hygiene has never been more important.

"Did you know there is at least 0.1 gram of faecal matter in the average pair of underwear of a toilet paper user?"

If you think 0.1 grams doesn't seem like much, do you realise that equates to 100 million E. coli bacteria floating around in their washing machine? If five underpants are in the wash, then make that 500 million E. coli bacteria floating around among the blouses, and handkerchiefs.

Perhaps many female teens are aware of this fact, hence why you use more toilet paper than males. Plus females care more about preventing skid marks in their underpants than males according to my research.

So What Other Uses Do Female Teens Have For Toilet Paper?

I wanted to find out the reason female teens use so much toilet paper, so I carried out a survey and also did some research among my customers and network. Here are some of the reasons I found:

- Females can't / don't shake dry.
- Females are more concerned about being hygienic. Menstruation needs.
- Soaking the toilet paper with water before wiping. Dry wiping a number 2 is disgusting.
- Using toilet paper for make-up removal, and wiping extra make up off.
- To fix make-up, like blot lipstick. To smudge eye shadow if I can't find my brush.
- Using toilet paper as a substitute for Kleenex. Clean off the outside of make-up containers.

- To remove runny makeup after sweating and crying (raccoon eyes).
- Cleaning up excess water around the sink.
- Using toilet paper to dry your hands when there are no hand towels in the bathroom.
- Females just need the toilet more than men, weaker bladders.
- Cleaning the toilet seat before sitting down (some guys have better aim than others).
- Padding the seat when it's cold and not your bathroom.
- To mop up sweat (the cleavage is sometimes sweaty).
- To absorb excessive applications of essential oil which I use instead of mist for perfume.
- We have much more to wipe up and many guys have revolting skid marks in their   underwear because you don't use enough.
- Fill my ears when my little brother won't be quiet.

What Harmful Chemicals Are Used In Toilet Paper?

With all this toilet paper use, is it perfectly safe? Excessive chemicals seem to be in everything these days. Well, one other huge benefit of The Bum Gun bidet sprayer which you might not be aware of is that you are saving your body from potentially harmful chemicals used in the manufacture of toilet paper.

Just one of the dangerous chemicals used in toilet paper is BPA (or byphenol A) that has been implicated in a number of illnesses, from prostate and breast cancer to hyperactivity in boys, as well as an increase in the risk of miscarriages. BPA rubs off easily onto the skin, especially into the sensitive skin around the rectum.
The National Institute of Environmental Health Sciences and the National Toxicology Program are concerned for the effects on the brain, behaviour, and the prostate gland in foetuses, infants, and children due to exposure to bisphenol A.

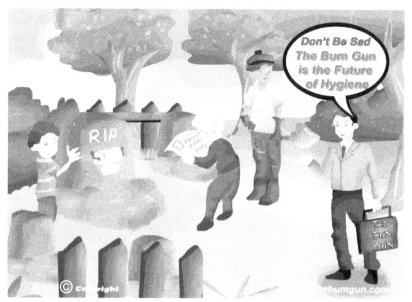

The Death of Toilet Paper

Prevention against chemicals in our lives should be important to everyone. Every time we reduce chemicals we are improving the quality of our lives, and reducing the chances of cancer.

What other chemicals are present in toilet paper which might act as an irritant or allergen?

I've carried out extensive research of the toilet paper industry so you don't have to and found that toilet paper, as well as facial tissues and paper towels contain formaldehyde. Formaldehyde is used in the toilet paper industry to improve the wet-strength and other "valued" characteristics of their products. For example, thick, absorptive, and white toilet paper is much more likely to contain formaldehyde than thinner, less expensive, duller, and more fragile types of paper.

Most people in the west currently think toilet paper is a "can't do without" personal hygiene product, and it is assumed that it contains no harmful chemicals. However, formaldehyde not only causes irritation, but it is also listed as a cancer-causing agent.

While, there are more than 100,000 chemicals used in commercial products, few have been tested for possible risks to health, yet those risks can be considerable. Surely it is common sense to do our best to the limit the exposure we and our families face in this chemicalized world.

Is White Toilet Paper Really Toxic?

Unfortunately yes. Have you ever wondered how toilet paper gets to be so white? The toilet paper industry has to use chlorine and chlorine dioxide to bleach it. This process creates cancer-causing chemicals such as dioxins and furans. Even low levels of exposure have been linked to many health problems such as cancer, hormone imbalances (dioxin is a hormone disruptor), immune system impairments, reduced fertility and birth defects. Dioxins cannot be excreted by our bodies, so they just accumulate over time. Many studies have found correlations between high exposure to dioxins and an increased risk of cancer.

To make the toilet paper white most pulp and paper mills use chlorine-based chemicals to bleach their pulp. These chemicals react with organic molecules in the wood and other fibres to create many toxic by-products, including dioxin. Dioxin is one of the most toxic human-made chemicals. Once released into the environment, it is persistent because natural bacteria cannot effectively break it down.

The Environmental Protection Agency has determined that using bleached toilet paper can result in a lifetime exposure to dioxin that exceeds acceptable risks. The FDA has also detected dioxins and dozens of other substances in conventional tampons and sanitary napkins. Chlorinated toilet paper also contains the highest amount of furans out of all cosmetic tissues.

The true issue with the amount of toilet paper used by female teens is that you are looking for a higher quality of cleaning yourself. There are many changes going on with your body with many issues to deal with, such as your menstruation. Therefore, it is perfectly right that you should be using more toilet paper than you used to. However, if you have a bidet sprayer installed you can save on toilet paper by anywhere between 80 and 100%. Perhaps you won't eradiate your need for toilet paper, but at least you can greatly reduce your use of it. Toilet paper will always be good for mopping up spills. While most users of a bidet sprayer use a towel to dry themselves, in a public bathroom that is not an option, so toilet paper is useful. In addition, your parents will also be very happy that your family shopping bill will reduce every month if your family invests in The Bum Gun, the 21st century answer to personal hygiene needs.

About Puberty and Your Body's Changes

Puberty is a special time in a girl's life because it means that you are growing up. But puberty can also be a very scary time in your life. Your body is going through changes, and your emotions are all over the place.

If you are going through puberty, you may be wondering if you are normal and this is something that a lot of girls wonder. Your body is going through a lot of changes and you may be wondering what it's all about. Here are some things that you should know about puberty.

Puberty Introduction

Puberty usually starts between the ages of 8 and 13 and will go on for a few years. Sometimes girls who are overweight start sooner and sometimes girls who are thin or very athletic start later. If you're 12 and your breasts haven't started developing or you're 15 and you haven't got your periods, you may want to see a doctor.
While going through puberty, your body is releasing hormones that stimulate the ovaries to begin producing estrogen, a female hormone. As time goes by, your body begins changing into that of a woman. However, these hormones also can make you moody, and sometimes you may feel that your body's going crazy.

Thoughts and Feelings During Puberty

1. Overly Sensitive

When you are going through puberty, your body is going through a lot of changes. That's why it's very common if you feel uncomfortable about these changes and be really sensitive about the way you look. Because of this, you might become easily irritated, feel depressed, or become angry easily. It's going to be useful to know the changes in the way you are acting and speak with someone about the way you feel.

2. Searching for Your Identity

Because you are turning into an adult, you might feel like you want to decide what is going to make you unique. A lot of girls your age also associate with their friends rather than the members of their family. This could be due to the fact that your friends are going through the same things that you are. You might try deciding how you're different from the other people and how you're fitting in. This could lead to a struggle to gain your independence from your family and parents.

3. Uncertainty

Because you're not totally an adult yet, but you're also not a child, you can feel uncertain about your life. This transitional phase may make you start wondering and thinking about unfamiliar and new things in your life like marriage, livelihood, and a career. Since it's all unfamiliar and new to start thinking about, you may feel like your future is uncertain.

This becomes much more evident when the people around you have more expectations about what you need to do. You might suddenly feel you have more responsibilities at home than a few years ago. Eventually you are going to grow into these new roles and gain more certainty about yourself. However, this process is going to take some time depending on your responses to the situations.

Peer Pressure

As you go through puberty, you are going to have a lot more conversations with your friends. You will likely be influenced by the things that you see around you in the media. Your friends and you may feel as if you want to try some of the things like alcohol and drugs. You also might want to dress and talk the way that the people you see are talking and dressing.

This could be uncomfortable sometimes and can even change what you like and dislike. It is also one way you may be struggling to be a part of your group. These kinds of events can also lead to gaps in between what's thought to be appropriate by your friends and your parents.

4. Conflicting Thoughts

Because you're in between being a child and an adult while going through puberty, you might feel stuck in life. An example would be that you want to have more independence but you are still looking for parental support. Another example might be whether you want to give up the things you loved doing when you were young so that you fit in with friends.

5. Mood Swings

Adding to the conflicting thoughts and uncertainty, you might also experience often and sometimes very extreme mood swings. Sometimes you are going to find that you are feeling happy and confident and then the next minute you are feeling depressed and irritated. These swings are very normal during puberty, and they happen because of hormone level shifts and other kinds of changes that you are going through.

6. Growing & Gaining Weight

Usually you will experience a few growth spurts in the beginning of puberty, while boys usually grow taller later. That's why you are going to notice that you are taller than most of the boys during your middle school years.

You are also going to notice that you are gaining weight. You may notice that you have more body fat. This is very normal. Don't diet unless your doctor tells you that you need to. This fat isn't bad. You need to have this fat for your menstrual cycle and your overall reproductive health. If you are unsure, get a second opinion from a gym instruction, your school sports teacher or another professional.

7. Breast Development

One thing that a lot of girls notice is that their breasts are growing, along with their hips becoming curvier. Inside your breasts, milk ducts develop so that you can breastfeed a baby someday. Their developing breasts are what often will stress girls out most about puberty. You may worry that your breasts aren't big enough. The thing to remember is that your breasts keep growing until you are 17, 18, or even when you're in your 20s. Sometimes one breast will grow slower than the other, though the other will usually catch up.

You will also notice changes in your nipples. They might become dark brown or pink, turned out or turned in. sometimes you will notice hairs around your nipples, too. This is perfectly normal.

If you want an idea about what you should expect about your breasts, it's a good idea to look at your mum. Your breasts' final size is partly based on your genes. The size won't be exactly the same, since you have your dad's genes, too, but it's a good indicator.

8. Menstruation

A couple of years after you begin developing breasts, chances are you will get your period. This will usually last 2-8 days and will come every month, or every 21-35 days. It may be a while before your periods are completely regular, however.

Every month, your uterus' lining becomes thick with blood so that an egg that's fertilized has a place to grow. When you aren't pregnant, this lining sheds and the blood is expelled from your vagina. Even though it seems like a lot, there's actually only a couple tablespoons of blood that are released.

9. Vaginal Discharge

It's possible that you are noticing white, sticky stuff inside your underwear. This is the fluid which helps keep your vagina clean and moist. Vaginal discharge often becomes stickier and thicker during your cycle. This discharge has a slight smell but it's undetectable by most people. Regular bathing using soap can help with reducing this odour, or of course using a bidet sprayer. In fact, regular users of a bidet sprayer often say the ability to have all day freshness around their vagina is one of the biggest, most important benefits of a bidet sprayer.

If your discharge becomes irritated or dry, is strong smelling, or is greenish or dark yellow, this can be a sign of an infection. You should see a doctor.

10. Body Hair

Another big thing that happens while you are going through puberty is the surprising growth of hair in strange places. You are going to notice it in your lower regions, your underarms, and even sometimes above your lips. Your leg and arm hair also often becomes thicker or darker.

Pubic hair generally starts with a couple of straight strands before becoming darker and curlier as it grows. Eventually it will become a triangle over your pubic bone and sometimes spreads to the inside of your thighs. The time when this starts is different for everyone – sometimes it's at the beginning, sometimes towards the end of puberty. If you find hair on your chin or chest, it's good to see a doctor. This might mean your hormones are off balance and this needs correction.

11. Sweating During Puberty

During puberty, you're going to find that you're sweating more. When bacteria and sweat combine, it leads to body odour. To control this odour, you want to ensure you are showering or bathing daily using a deodorant soap and also antiperspirant under your arm. The antiperspirants with a lot of aluminium chloride are stronger than the other ones. If you find a rash beneath your arms, it's possible you're allergic to aluminium and you should find one that doesn't have it in it. It's also a good idea to choose fabrics with moisture wicking material since they are going to dry much faster and you won't have to worry about armpit stains as much.

It's possible that your feet will also get sweaty. Wearing cotton socks will help with absorbing moisture. It's also important to wear different shoes so that your shoes can dry. Don't wear plastic, rubber, or other types of manmade materials.

My mum was always so serious about only buying leather shoes when I was a teenager. We often had mini-battles when I saw a pair of awesome shoes, but they turned out to be fake leather. She was always so insistent that all my shoes had to be real leather. I didn't realize how smart she was at the time. Later though I understood when many of my friends would develop foot problems, such as smelly feat and rotten skin because their fake leather shoes did not allow their feet to breathe.

12. Problems With Acne

Another problem with puberty is the appearance of acne. These are whiteheads, pimples, and blackheads and they are due to your hormones surging. If acne is a problem, try using a non-soap cleanser and acne products that have salicylic acid or benzoyl peroxide in them. These don't require a prescription. Also look for moisturizers, makeup, and sunscreen that have non-comedogenic or oil free on the labels. If you are still having problems, you might want to see a dermatologist. Also, please see chapter 4 where there is a lot more information on acne.

Puberty Conclusion

You are going through many things physically and you have a lot of emotions going through you. Remember that everything is normal and that these things will pass. Your body is doing what it needs to do to turn you into an adult. You are going through what your parents and their parents went through, and you will get through it. If you find that you need to talk to someone, try talk to someone at school or talk to a trusted relative, your sister or parents.

Tips For Personal Hygiene During Menstruation

Your personal hygiene needs change once you become a teenager, and also change as you move through your teen years. Therefore, personal hygiene is something that you should always keep in mind. When you start to have your periods, having good personal hygiene is very important. Learning the menstrual hygiene basics helps to make sure that you are well informed about the proper way to remain healthy and steer clear of infections during menstruation.

Menstruation is one time that a lot of women have problems with infections, including infections that are sexually transmitted. Even if you aren't sexually active, learning good personal hygiene practices at a young age can help you with creating good habits for later in life. You are at greater risk of developing an infection during your period since the mucus, which is usually blocking your cervix, opens up during menstruation. This allows the blood to come out of your body. Because of this, bacteria also can travel into your pelvic cavity and your uterus. Changes in your vaginal pH can also make your chance of developing a yeast infection more likely.

It's essential that you understand the right practices for personal period hygiene and the situations and actions which will put you at risk so that you are able to maintain a menstrual routine that is best for your overall health.

Best Practices for Good Hygiene During Menstruation

Bathe Regularly

When you have your period, one of the best things that you can do is to bathe morning and night. This is going to help keep your body smelling good and keep it clean. You should also wash your hands properly when you go to the bathroom, before and after you clean your vagina, and before and after when changing your pad or tampon.

Wash Your Body Correctly

Your vagina is a very sensitive area and it's more sensitive than other areas on your body. It will require a different type of wash. It's best to wash your vagina on the outside and you should never use regular soap, shampoo, or douches on your vaginal area. These can upset your natural acidity and flora. Instead, use a soap that's specially created for using on your intimate area or simply use warm water and your hand.

Wear The Right Clothing

We know that you love wearing tight pants that you think are cute, but these can negatively affect your vagina's health. Wearing clothing that's tight can lead to increased heat and moisture, along with irritating your skin. It's better to choose cotton underwear and clothing that is loose fitting. This will lead to a healthier vagina.

Change Your Sanitary Items Often

You should change a sanitary towel for a new one approximately every four hours, during the day, even if the flow of blood is not very great. This will make you feel cleaner and is better for you. If you continually use the same tampon or pad, it increases the risk that you have of TSS and infection. TSS stands for toxic shock syndrome, which is a very serious infection which can land you in the hospital. Another problem with going too long between changing pads is that your skin can become irritated, and this can lead to broken skin and a higher risk of infection.

Use the Correct Absorbency of Tampon

When using tampons, it's important to choose the lowest absorbency necessary for your menstrual flow. And because the amount of flow varies from day to day, it's likely that you will need to use different absorbencies on different days of your period. Selecting the right absorbency comes with experience, but use this as a guide.

Note: If a tampon absorbs as much as it can and has to be changed before 4 hours, then you may want to try a higher absorbency. On the other hand, if you remove a tampon and after 4-8 hours white fibre is still showing, you should choose a lower absorbency. When using a tampon at night for up to 8 hours, choose the lowest absorbency needed, insert a fresh one just before going to bed and remove it as soon as you wake up in the morning.

If you are using tampons rather than pads, you should always use the lowest absorbency possible for your flow. You should also never use a tampon when you aren't menstruating. Using the super absorbent tampons when you are only lightly bleeding can greatly increase your TSS risk.

Toilet Paper vs. the Bidet Sprayer

For far too long females have been restricted by what they can use to keep their private areas clean between showers. Fortunately, there have been some fantastic developments in bathroom hygiene in the last few years. Obviously both sexes care about personal hygiene, but arguably females need a more advanced and efficient way to clean throughout the day.

The bidet sprayer is basically a miniature shower hose which is installed right next to the toilet. Unlike, the traditional bidets where you had to hop off onto another device, the bidet sprayer can be used

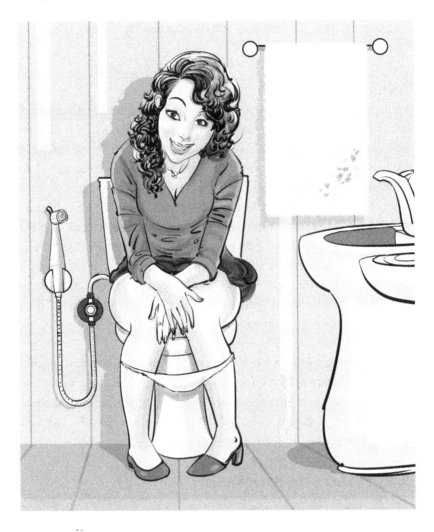

while you are sitting on the toilet which is much more convenient, and bidet sprayers are much cheaper in the long run.

The bidet sprayer is basically used instead of toilet paper to clean your private parts after a no.2, after urination and whenever you need to change your pad or tampon during menstruation. I really feel sorry for anyone who has not been lucky enough to experience this innovation in personal hygiene. And I promise you one thing today, you will never go back to toilet paper, after experiencing the awesome clean the bidet sprayer gives you.

I'm not joking or exaggerating when I say no one goes back to toilet paper after discovering The Bum Gun. This is a mighty impressive fact that you should remember.

Don't make the mistake of believing a few people on the Internet who don't know what they are talking about. I'll tell you a true story you'll find shocking. On one forum discussing bidet sprayers versus toilet paper, there was someone who actually thought that using water to clean after the toilet was "disgusting". Honestly, that's no lie. Just goes to show what numbskulls there can be on the Internet spouting all sorts of rubbish.

A Little Thing to Change What You Mean by Clean

I saw an advertisement the other day for Andrex Washlets that made me laugh. These pre-moistened wipes are as they say "a little extra step to your existing routine". And by 'little' I suppose they are right. But why take a little step in being cleaner after using the toilet? Why not take a huge step and get "shower fresh clean" with water? If you want to be properly clean, use the soothing water jet of The Bum Gun bidet sprayer every time.

Are Wet Wipes Flushable?

The manufacturers say these wet wipes are flushable. But that is not what water authority companies inform us. They say wet toilet tissues like Andrex Washlets are not environmentally friendly because when they're flushed down the toilet they take longer to break down. One water company is spending upwards of £12 million a year on asking their staff to get down into the sewers and shovel the gunk out. Do you think the water companies are going to ride these added costs, or pass them on to all of us? Of course they are going to pass on the costs of clearing all these blockages to all of us. The need to feel clean is a very natural and commendable one. And my presumption for people's choice of wet wipes is a natural development from the age old toilet paper. These people just haven't discovered the bum gun bidet sprayer yet.

One article I read in a newspaper was hounding users of wet wipes for trying to be cleaner and more hygienic, accusing consumers of buying "pointless feminine hygiene products". The journalist's point, who was no other than Janet Street Porter no less (she's actually quite famous in the UK), was just to stick with toilet paper. She questioned why females, but could equally have said anyone, would not be satisfied with toilet paper, and looked for a cleaner option. It's abundantly clear to me that either Ms Porter doesn't think personal hygiene is important, prefers to live in the dark ages or is ignorant of the developments in bathroom hygiene and bidet sprayers in particular over the last few years. Perhaps I should send the poor dear our best-selling bidet sprayer.

I'd also like to educate Ms Porter on some environmental issues. She shouts down wet wipes as not being environmentally sound, but clearly doesn't know the massive production processes of toilet paper either.

So if you want to be properly clean between pad changes and using the toilet, think about trying The Bum Gun bidet sprayer after every bathroom visit.

> *"One senses that no amount of wet-wiping*
> *could bring true hygiene."*
> **— Tahir Shah, Travels With Myself**

Benefits of The Bum Gun In Brief
- Will help you avoid hand contamination from normal wiping
- Provide a gentler form of cleansing after the toilet or during menstruation
- Prevent pain on your tender bits from abrasive toilet paper
- Help you prevent soiled underwear and uncleanliness
- Have a cleansing, soothing, and refreshing feeling after every bathroom visit

- Help you avoid using potentially irritating feminine hygiene sprays and deodorants
- Help avoid some of the irritation of haemorrhoids that toilet paper can cause
- And of course decrease your exposure to chemicals which can never be underestimated, with cancer rates expected to increase by 50% to 15 million new cases by 2020, according to the World Cancer Report, the most comprehensive global examination of the disease to date

No Bidet Sprayer in the Bathroom?

When you are in a bathroom without a bidet sprayer - Wipe Starting at the Front: When you wipe from your back to your front, you are risking exposing yourself to harmful bacteria from your anal region. This can lead to infections like urinary tract and yeast. It's also a good idea to cleanse your anal and vaginal areas separately.

You want to make sure that you stay clean and healthy down there using the correct hygienic procedures. Otherwise you are going to feel sick and possibly get an infection, and you likely won't smell good either.

FAQ About Menstruation

If you have just started getting your periods or you have had them for a while, you may have a few questions that you are embarrassed to ask but you really want to know. Here are some common questions and answers to them.

At What Age Do Women Get Their First Period?

Most girls will get their period for the first time in between 11-14, but sometimes it will come sooner or later. There isn't a right age when girls start their periods. Talk to your mum and find out when she got hers the first time. This can give you a good indication of when you are going to get your period.

How Can I Alleviate My Cramps?

When you have your period, you can help alleviate cramp pain by taking a bath. You also can wear comfy sweats and simply relax. You also can use OTC medications, yoga, meditation, or a heating pad, like a hot water bottle on your stomach. It also helps if you stay away from spicy or greasy foods.

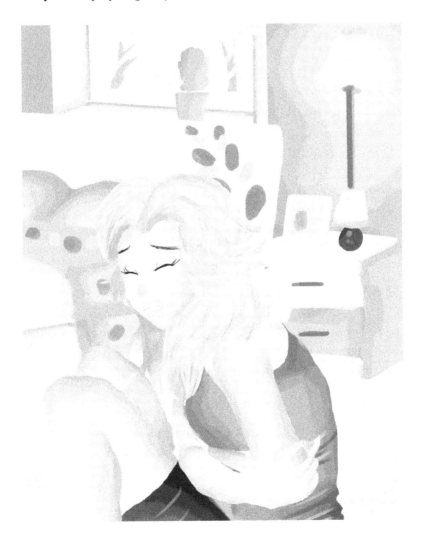

How Do I Know My Period Is Coming?

There are a few signs that your period is coming, and they're different for everybody. It will be a lot easier once you're older and you get to know your body, but some things that might happen are:

- Your breasts and back hurt
- You become constipated
- You're hungry but bloated
- You get depressed and/or irritable easily
- Your face gets spots

My Period's Brown Not Red, Is This Normal?

This is completely normal and it often happens when your period starts and ends. This just means that the fluid's leaving your body slower. It's brown because it has more time to oxidize. The rest of your blood turns brown once it's been out in the air a while.

How Long Should My Period Last?

This fluctuates but usually a period lasts from 2-6 days. This includes a day or two of heavy flow when your period starts and then a couple of days when you will have a lighter flow. The amount that you are menstruating can vary and that's completely normal.
The following are signs you should look for:

- Changing sanitary product more often than once an hour
- Steady stream that won't stop
- Period lasting longer than a week

If you are noticing these things, you should see a doctor.

Is It Possible To Delay My Period Or Stop It?

There isn't a natural way that you can change your period's start day or stop it quicker. There are a few birth control pills that are able to make your period come only a couple of times per year, but they aren't safe for every woman and they have a few side effects. If you want to try a birth control pill, you should speak with your mum and then your doctor.

My Periods Are Irregular, What Does That Mean?

Most cycles are approximately 28 days, but women have different cycles. Your schedule may change between months because of sickness, weight change, or stress. For the first two years following your first period, you are likely to have irregular periods. Sometimes you might even skip a month. This can be very scary, especially if you are sexually active. But if you aren't sexually active, and especially if you have recently started getting your period, chances are that you are just irregular. If you are concerned, talk to someone you trust about it.

Can I Get Pregnant When I Have My Period?

A lot of women think that they can't get pregnant while they are having their period, but this is a myth. Anytime you have unprotected sex, you are able to get pregnant.

My Period's Late. Help!

Don't start freaking out. As mentioned above, your period can fluctuate. If you have had vaginal sex, it's a good idea to go and get a test. This can be purchased in a store if you don't want to go to the doctor. But it may be that you are just late and have nothing to worry about.

How Accurate Are Home Pregnancy Tests?

A home pregnancy test kit will measure the level of a hormone called, human chorionic gonadotropin (or hCG for short). Non-pregnant women do not have this hormone in their body. Most home pregnancy test kits are fairly accurate, with most claiming 99% accuracy. But there is a problem if you take a home pregnancy test too early. You may get a negative result even when you are definitely pregnant. For some women, it takes them a while before the amount of hCG in their urine is high enough for a home pregnancy test to pick it up. For this reason, you should take more tests again if you have missed a period and don't know if you're pregnant or not.

What's Spotting and Why Is It Happening To Me?

Spotting is a light flow of blood in between the time of your periods. It doesn't happen to every woman and although it isn't harmful, it's often annoying. If you have spotting, it's a good idea to use a panty liner when you notice the spotting happening.

Which Is Better – Tampons Or Pads?

Many women like using tampons better because they're much more discreet. Plus, they are great for the summer months since you can go swimming using them. But it's all a personal choice as to which is more comfortable for you.

We have added a useful glossary at the back of the book for detailed descriptions of any potentially confusing vocabulary.

Greg & Cristina Noland

Chapter 3
Natural Beauty Tips & Makeup Ideas

"Mum, can I wear makeup to school!" These words will probably strike fear into most mothers when they first hear them, as to your mum it feels like only yesterday when she was preparing your packed lunch box and walking you to school.

So what is the right age for you to wear makeup, to school, or even at all? I think the golden rule here, is to take your time. Many girls might start with some lip gloss between 10 and 12, and then wish to advance to mascara and a bit of foundation around the 13 to 14 mark. But all parents are different, as well as the desires of the teenagers.

But whenever you are allowed to start wearing makeup, you are going to want to have the advice from the experts. Therefore, I have teamed up with some of the best makeup specialists I could find to help me write this chapter. Let's dive straight in to some really useful information.

How Much Does Beauty Impact Our Lives?

You don't have to move very far every day until you are bombarded by advertisements for hair, skin, teeth, and make-up. Pick up any magazine and you are bound to find at least a few advertisements for a wonder diet, low fat foods, and memberships to gyms. You could say we are all fairly excessive about our looks. But how much does our beauty impact our lives? I would go as far to say the myth of female beauty challenges every woman, every day of her life. It doesn't matter if she at school or university, in the media, in relation-ships between men and women, and between women and women, the pressure to look good is everywhere. Are women consumed by this potentially destructive obsession? Does putting so much effort into our beauty really give us a better quality of life?

It is my feeling that we all put much more importance on looks than we care to admit. But with the right tips and advice, we don't need to let the pressure to look good consume us. As a teenager, you will be curious about beauty and the things that you can do to make yourself look great. You are probably curious about shaving, makeup, hair, and lots of other things that you have only heard about up until now. Therefore, this chapter will give you some simple, yet effective advice for looking your best, with the minimum of fuss.

Let's take a look at what this section on beauty will cover.

- Natural beauty tips
- Beauty substitutions
- Shaving
- Eyebrows
- Skin tips
- Hair / Nails / Makeup

Natural Beauty Tips

Before we get into the makeup that you buy in the store, we're going to take a look at some of the natural treatments that you can use to make yourself look beautiful.

Avocados

You may know avocado as something that's yummy in guacamole and that tastes great on tacos and burritos. But there are a lot of other reasons that you should love avocado. Bet you didn't know that it's great to add into your beauty routine, too. It has a lot of benefits for your hair and your skin.

Here are a few reasons that you should think of avocado as something that's not just a side dish.

1. It is a great, all-natural moisturizer – The amazing avocado is filled with natural oils that are able to deeply go into your skin much better than a lot of products to keep your skin hydrated and soft. Just mash up one of your avocados and put it right onto your body and face. Allow it to stay there for a few minutes and then jump into the shower. This might sound weird but you'll love the way your skin feels.

2. It is great for your cuticles – Get an avocado the next time you're at your store. When you are doing your nails the next time, use it on your cuticles. They will feel soft and it will make your hands soft too.

3. It helps you glow – Since they're filled with carotenoids and antioxidants, they help improve your skin's overall appearance. Want a great facemask? Cut an avocado in half and mash half of it, then mix in ¼ teaspoon honey. Put it on your skin and leave it 10 minutes, then use a dampened cloth to rinse off.

4. It helps with preventing blackouts and reduces scars from acne – Avocados are full of Vitamins E, and that's a big in-gredient in a lot of acne treatments. It also helps with reducing acne scars. Use the mask above once per week and you'll see a difference.

5. It is great for conditioning damaged, dry hair – Is your hair damaged? Or do you just want it to be shinier? Avocados are great for this! Whisk together one egg yolk, a teaspoon of honey, and one teaspoon of olive oil. Then, mash up half of an avocado and mix everything together. Put it on your hair, particularly on your ends, and allow it to sit for approximately 15 minutes. Rinse your hair off and shampoo it. You are going to be so surprised at the shiny, soft results.

6. It is great for soothing sunburns – Even though you always use sunscreen (wink, wink) sunburns can happen. Apply some avocado that you have mashed up and you'll get relief instantly.

Coconut Oil

You probably think of coconut as something that you smell when you slather on your suntan lotion or use your favourite body spray or shampoo. But the truth is that there are a lot of benefits that you will find when you're incorporating coconut oil into your beauty routine and everyday routine. .

1. **Natural deodorant** – Put coconut oil onto the spots where you have a lot of trouble with sweating. You also can make your own deodorant using coconut oil, baking soda, arrow-root, and shea butter.
2. **Remover for eye makeup** - Soak cotton with coconut oil and use it for removing waterproof, stubborn makeup.
3. **Hydrating conditioner** - Mix a cup of hot water and 2 tablespoons coconut oil (more if you have long hair). After the oil settles, massage it into your hair and scalp, comb your hair using a comb with wide teeth, put your hair up in a bun, and put on a shower cap. Allow it to sit for 60 minutes and then thoroughly rinse it using warm water to get beautiful, shiny hair.
4. **Cuticle cream** - Putting coconut oil right on your cuticles will help soften your cuticles and make your nails stronger.
5. **Exfoliator** - Mix 2 tablespoons sugar and 3 tablespoons coconut oil and leave it in a jar so that you have an exfoliator anytime you need it that will make your skin glow.
6. **Zipper fixer** - Put a swab into some coconut oil, then rub it onto a stuck zipper and it will come loose.
7. **Body moisturizer** - It helps with softening your skin and treating dry elbows and cracked heels.
8. **De-frizzer** - Put a bit of the oil on your hair and on its ends to make it sleek and shiny.
9. **Lip Balm** - Works wonders with healing chapped dry lips quickly.
10. **Sunburn soother** - Putting it onto sunburn will help with soothing and sealing it.

11. **Shaving cream** - Put some of this onto your legs and you are going to notice that you're feeling much smoother after shaving.

12. **Highlighter** - Once your makeup's on, put a little on your nose's bridge and your cheeks for beautifully glowing skin.

13. **Flyaway tamer -** When you massage this into your hair, you won't have problems with flyaways anymore.

14. **Face Mask -** Blend equal amounts raw honey and coconut oil and then put it right on your face. Allow it to sit 3-4 minutes and then use warm water to rinse it off. You will find glowing and really smooth skin underneath.

15. **Cleaner for makeup brushes** - Microwave 3-4 tablespoons coconut oil for approximately 30 seconds. When you bring it out, dip your makeup brushes into it. Take a napkin or paper towel and rub your brushes with it to take off the makeup. Finish up by rinsing the brushes with warm water. Because of the oil's anti-fungal benefits, it will help with keeping the brushes free of bacteria.

16. **Scar treatment -** The oil's antioxidants and Vitamin E help with healing scars and smoothing out your skin for a complexion that's clearer.

Beauty Substitutions

There are some times when you go to reach for something and you find that you are out. But the good news is that there are often some items that you can find around the house that you can use to substitute for your favourite beauty items. Here are some of the things that you can do when you find you have an emergency.

1. **Don't have polish remover? Perfume to the rescue!**
   Even though you probably think of perfume as something that you should put on your pulse points, you can use perfume for removing nail polish. A solvent that's contained in perfumes can help with removing the nail lacquer if you are in a bind. The same thing that is in perfume is also in polish removers that aren't acetone based. Put some

perfume onto a ball of cotton and then use it like you would a polish remover.

2. **Out of deodorant? Baking soda is great!**

There's nothing worse than being stinky because you don't have any deodorant. But you don't have to have this problem when you use some baking soda. It will break down and then neutralize those acids that cause the stinky body odour. Just mix it with some water and then rub it on.

3. **Don't have anything to remove your eye makeup? Use some organic coconut oil.**

You may not know this, but oils can help with breaking down waxy items like mascara, eye shadow, and eyeliner. The eye makeup removers that are most effective contain oils. So if you don't have any remover, get some coconut oil. This also has another perk. It works on waterproof makeup and it's gentle and can help condition your lashes.

4. **Don't have any primer? Aloe gel's a great option!**

Aloe's a great substitute for primer. It helps with hydrating and smoothing your skin's surface and minimizing pores. It also helps with keeping your makeup where it belongs and fresh looking. It's also great for people who have dry skin.

5. **Don't have eyeliner? Grab your mascara and angled brush**

Mascara's very similar to gel or cream liners in its formula and it can be used for eyeliner if you don't have one. If you want the best results, look for mascara that's waterproof since your oils in your eyelids won't break it down as easily. Just use some of the mascara from your wand with your angled brush and put it on like cream liners.

7. **Out of powder? Use some corn-starch**

Corn-starch will remove the shine and keeps the oil balance on your face. It also will ensure the longevity of your makeup and won't change your foundation's colour if it's correctly applied. Us a large brush and vigorously shake off any excess. (Try tapping your brush against something hard to make sure you have an application that is light.) Put a light dusting on your face and you are done. Remember that corn-starch is white, so it's the choice for people who have light complexions. If you have a darker complexion, you can mix it with cocoa powder until the shade is right.

8. **Out of bronzer? Cocoa powder is a great option**
   If you aren't allergic, you can use cocoa powder for a bronzer. Not only that but it smells wonderful. Put your powder into corn-starch bit by bit until you've reached the right shade. After you have found the right tone, use a bronzer brush just like any bronzer you bought in the store.

9. **Don't have moisturizer? Turn to the sheet masks**
   Chances are you have some of these somewhere in your room. These great masks are soaked with essence and contain the same types of antioxidants, vitamins, and other kinds of ingredients that are found in moisturizers and serums. They're so drenched that there is often a lot left in the packets. Drain the extra essences and then put it in your purse. You are going to have what you need anytime, anywhere. Tap this onto your cheekbones to give yourself a glow or use it after working out for flawless complexion.

Shaving Myths & Facts

Now that you have hair in places that you didn't have it before, you will want to start shaving. But before we look at the tips for shaving, let's look at some of the myths that you might believe about shaving:

Myth

When I begin shaving, I'll need to do it constantly, even when it's winter.

Fact

Shaving's basically just cutting the hair on your body really close to your skin. When you are shaving, you aren't changing your hair follicles or how it's growing. So it's okay to shave for the warm seasons and not do it when it's wintertime, if you don't want.

Myth

When I shave every day, my hair is going to grow back darker and thicker.

Fact

When you're shaving, you are simply cutting your hair's surface and everything beneath your skin's left alone. When your hair grows back at first, your hair might feel different since shaving will cut it on an angle. However, soon it's going to feel silky and soft like before you started shaving.

Myth

Shaving using soap or water alone is as good as when I use shaving cream.

Fact

Water and soap isn't good for getting close shaves. Soap's made to clean your skin and remove the oils as well as any dirt, which means your skin's vulnerable and dry. Water alone softens your hair and skin but it disappears too fast to help you with shaving.

Shaving gel gives a blanket which keeps your hair soft while you're shaving and it lubricates. This allows the razor to go much easier over the skin. Another good thing about shaving gel is that it isn't going to clog razors like soap.

Myth

It's okay if I dry shave once in a while.

Fact

It's never a good idea to dry shave. If you are going out in a mini skirt or you are going to the pool, take a few minutes to properly shave. A couple of minutes soaking the hair in some warm water and then applying shave cream is going to help you avoid razor burn and painful cuts and nicks. If you do dry shaving, though, it can make you not want to go out in shorts because you could have embarrassing scabs and scrapes.

Myth

It's only necessary to shave my pits when I'm not wearing sleeves.

Fact

Removing the hair from your pits isn't just about giving you silky, clean looking pits. Along with keeping you feeling fresh, removing the hair reduces the possibility of bacteria build-up, the biggest reason for armpit odour.

Myth

Using a new razor will give me a lot more cuts and nicks. It's important to break in my razor.

Fact

This isn't true – it's actually the opposite. Shaving using a blade that's dull can lead to cuts and nicks. A fresh, sharp razor which has at least three blades is going to give you a closer, cleaner shave and you are going to have less chance of cutting yourself while shaving.

Myth

I can get a better, closer shave when I press hard.

Fact

Using a touch that's light with a sharp, clean, fresh razor is the best way to get skin that's silky smooth. Be very careful and use a light hand on areas such as knees, bikini area, and ankles.

Myth
Shaving will make my skin flaky and dry.
Fact

Not true at all. When you shave with razors, it will actually help your skin feel and look smoother because it removes your skin's dead cells on the top, particularly if you're using shave gel or cream and you're shaving after you shower. Use moisturizer after shaving for skin that's even silkier.

Myth
My tan will fade faster if I shave.
Fact

It's impossible to shave off a tan. Tanning's the function of your skin producing melanin. Shaving will actually enhance a tan because it removes the flaky skin layers that often hide the tan's glow.

Myth
Shaving my sensitive areas, like my bikini line, will always make me itchy and cause bumps.
Fact

Shaving your sensitive areas doesn't need to leave your bikini bumpy and itchy. For a shave that's silky smooth all the time, condition your hair and skin before you shave with a bath or shower and shave using a shaving gel that contains moisturizer.

When you are shaving, pull your skin back so the areas flat and firm. Use gentle strokes and a very light touch, going in a comfortable direction. Lots of shave gel and a fresh razor will let you use less pressure. If you need to go back over an area, use more gel before continuing.

After you have finished shaving, rinse using cold water so your pores are closed. Pat the skin dry and then apply a little powder to give you a fresh, cool feeling.

Shaving Mistakes to Avoid

Doing your shaving right when you get in the shower

You may want to do this first thing in the morning and as soon as you get in the shower, but it's a better idea to wait 15 minutes before beginning to shave. This is going to soften your hair and help your follicles to open up. But don't wait longer than 15 minutes because your skin will swell and wrinkle, meaning your shave won't be as close. Plus it is not a good idea to shave in the shower with the water running as you will waste a lot of water.

Doing it before school

If you shave at night, your legs will be smoother longer. While you are sleeping, your legs are going to swell slightly, which may make your hair retreat back into the follicles.

Not lathering up or using a bar of soap

Even if you're really in a hurry, you shouldn't dry shave. Use a moisturizing shaving cream to be sure your razor will easily glide over your legs and this will avoid cuts and nicks. If you don't have shaving cream, you can use hair conditioner. But don't use a bar of soap. It doesn't give you the lubrication you need.

Using disposable razors with one blade

This is okay if you do it occasionally, but you shouldn't use them every day. Choose a razor that has four or five blades. They give you the smoothest shave and let you go over the hard areas like your ankles and knees.

Not replacing razors blades often

You might have bought a good razor but if you don't buy new blades when the old ones become dull, it won't do you any good. A blade will usually last anywhere from 5-10 shaves

Shaving up before shaving down

When you are doing your first sweep, shave in your hair growth's direction which is down your leg. If you have problems with sensitive skin, don't shave up your leg ever. Even though going upward might give you a shave that's closer, it increases the chances that you will have irritation, cuts, and nicks. After your hair is short and your skin's lubricated and warm, going down will be a lot safer. Don't forget to use more gel before doing that second pass.

Not treating or preventing razor burn

Shaving close often leads to ingrown hairs. Not treating razor burn often can lead to scars that will stay around. To help with preventing red bumps, use a body scrub that exfoliates twice per week to get rid of the skin that's trapping the hairs. To treat the bumps, place warm compresses on the area that's affected. That heat will relax your hair. After you have showered, put lotion on your skin to soften your hair. This will leave your skin much less infection prone.

Eyebrow Maintenance

You may not be up to this point in your beauty regime, but when you are, it's good to know what to do and what not to do when it comes to your eyebrows. Let's dive straight in with some of the mistakes to avoid by some leading eyebrow experts.

Mistakes to Avoid

Over plucking

Plucking eyebrows daily is something that some people find satisfying, but the professionals say it's not a good idea. According to Santi Garay and Michelle Wu, two eyebrow specialists, it's best to tweeze your eyebrows once every 21 days. This is because the hairs that grow differently have the time to grow, and therefore your brows are going to look much more even.

Using old tweezers

If you find that hairs are going through the tweezers or you can't bring your points together, you need new tweezers. You also shouldn't allow the tweezers to become gunky in your bag of makeup. Use isopropyl alcohol to clean them before and after using them so that bacteria doesn't build up.

Don't overdo the sides

Try to steer clear of unibrows as there are many women who over pluck in between the brows. This is going to make your nose look bigger and your eyes really far apart. The beginning of your eyebrows should align with the bridge of your nose, not the outer edge of your nostrils. Don't over pluck your outer brows, either. So that you can determine where your eyebrows should end, picture a line that goes diagonally from the corner of your nose to the outside corner of your eye. You can use something like a pencil to guide you.

Making a huge arch

Paisley or rainbow shaped brows make you look constantly surprised. So that you can find your arch, look for the highest point of your eyebrow, which is usually around 2/3 of the way from the inside of your brow (it shouldn't be centred perfectly). Tweeze below your brow so that you have a lift. If your brows are lighter in colour, you can use brow powder to darken your shape before you pluck so that you're able to see. Then just pluck around your shape but don't overdo it.

Forgetting about the top

Tweezing below your brow creates a lovely lift but you should remember about the top. Keep your above-brow area completely free of the stray hairs, since they are much more noticeable in that area.

Overusing the eyebrow pencil

If you just put a few feathery strokes on your brow using your eyebrow pencil, it's going to take your eyebrows from just so-so to well-defined and amazing. Choose a pencil that's one shade lighter compared with your eyebrows' colour. When your brow is really dark, they look fake and harsh. Use some light strokes so that you can shade in the patchy sections and then trace your brows' natural shape. If you aren't comfortable using a pencil, you can use a brush on an angle that's been dipped in some brow powder that is lighter than your natural colour.

Take Advantage of a Pro

If you aren't sure about the way that your brow looks or how it should look, or if you have made a mistake that needs fixing, you can go see a professional. Even if this is only 1-2 times each year, they will help you find your brow's natural shape and they can also give you some expert guidelines for your own routine. Your eyebrows give your eyes attention and make them your face's focal point. Therefore they are very important to your appearance.

Advice on Nails

Chances are that you, and a lot of your friends, wear nail polish on your fingernails and your toenails. So we know how important it is to you to have some tips and tricks to make them look great. So this section is dedicated to your nails.

Tips for Keeping Your Nails Healthy

Don't constantly wear polish on your nails

When you have nail polish on every day it can cause yellowing of your nails. If your nails are discoloured, mix a tablespoon baking soda, a half of a teaspoon olive oil, and some lemon juice. Rub it into your finger and toenails and let it sit for ten minutes. Then rinse the mixture off. Your nails are going to look incredibly clean. Give your nails a break from the polish every couple of weeks to stop the stains.

Don't cut the cuticles

Hangnails often are caused when cuticles are cut too much. If you go and get a manicure, let the technician know that you just want them pushed back. You can also use some cuticle or coconut oil on them so they stay healthy.

Don't use polish remover with acetone in it

Acetone will strip away the natural oils in your nails. This will make them dry and therefore they will likely break more often. Look for a formula that doesn't have acetone in it.

Never pick at your chipped polish

Anytime your polish is chipping, you are also losing a nail layer. When you notice your manicure and pedicure coming off, simply remove it rather than picking the polish off. You can avoid having chips altogether by putting top coats on whenever you polish.

Don't skip your base coat

Are you one of those girls who hate nail ridges anytime you don't have polish on? The good news is that wearing base coat will help. It fills the ridges in. To make your nails stronger, look for one that has calcium in it.

Remember to give your nails moisture

Nails are made from keratin, and this needs moisture to grow healthy. Now here is a really neat trick I learnt from a supermodel. Slather some heavy cream upon your feet and hands before you go to bed, and wear gloves and socks on your hands and feet to lock that moisture in and help to heal your nails.

Choose the right time to trim your nails

Your nails are going to be less breakable and softer after you take a shower. You can also cut them anytime your nails are soft, like after you have washed the dishes.

Don't file your nail's surface

If you file their surfaces, your nails will become thin. Rather than doing this, use your buffer on the nail's surface and stick to filing the edges.

Hand and Nail Care ContainingTriclosan

Avoid soaps and hand sanitizers that contain the harsh chemical triclosan (often marked "antibacterial") which is the main antibacterial ingredient in many non-alcoholic hand sanitizers.

According to the Public Health Agency of Canada (PHAC), and the World Health Organization (WHO) hand sanitizers that contain between 60 and 80 percent alcohol are "an excellent" way to clean your hands when you're not near a sink. But be careful, high amounts of alcohol can dehydrate your skin and nails, making your polish chip faster. Professional manicurists advise to moisturize your hands and nails after using hand sanitizers, just remember to wait for the sanitizer to dry.

Never seesaw nails

File in just one direction. This will help to avoid splitting your nail-bed.

Don't grow really long nails

You may not know it, but if your nails are long they can carry a lot of harmful bacteria beneath them. These bacteria can lead vomiting and diarrhoea. Make sure that you cut and file your nails regularly. They are going to be healthier and they will also make life a lot easier too.

Tips for Finding the Right Nail Polish Shade for Your Skin Tone

Often as a teen you will have trouble choosing the right colour of nail polish for you, so here are some tips that you can use to find the right colour based on your skin tone.

1. Skin That's Really Fair

If you have really fair skin, you may have pink undertones in your skin. So here are some tips for finding the right nail polish colour for you.

Colours for you to try
- Wear the shades that are pastels.
- Really dark blue, midnight blue, and navy blue are great shades if you are interested in wearing dark shades.
- You are also able to wear dark pinks and reds.

Colours you need to avoid
- Don't wear black nail polish.
- It's not a good idea to wear polish colours with a lot of pink undertones.
- Don't use invisible or sheer colours since they have undertones that are going to blend complete with your skin.

2. Skin That's Fair

If you have fair skin, there are different light shades that you can try.

Colours for you to try
- Lots of different types of pastel colours.
- Ruby and dark red shades
- Purple, burgundy, and plums
- White, pale pinks, and silver
- Orange, blues, peach
- Don't wear any colours that are really dark with the exception of red.

3. Skin That's Medium

If your skin is medium toned, you can wear a lot of different types of colours easily.

Colours for you to try
- Light purples, pinks, reds, and blues
- Burgundy and silver
- Pale brown and peach

Colours you need to avoid

Don't wear any shades of rust and gold.

4. Skin That's Medium Dark

If your skin is medium dark, the deep shades are going to be the best for you.

Colours for you to try

Bright orange, red, and purples

Colours you need to avoid

Stay away from anything that's pastel or that is light in colour since it will make you look washed out.

Important Tips: This is a really useful tip often ignored by teenage girls. Even though it's really important that your nail polish complements the tone of your skin, it's equally essential that you choose colours that are based on what you are wearing and what the occasion is.

Along with this, make sure your nails are clean and that they are trimmed regularly which can also make your nails look more beautiful. And remember to wash your hands regularly throughout the day for best hand hygiene. Most people don't realize this but on average we all touch our eyes, nose, and mouth at least 16 times per hour whether you realise it or not. Also, on average people put their finger in their nose at least 5 times per hour. Hence the need to make sure you wash your hands regularly throughout the day.

Tips for Creating the Perfect at Home Pedi and Mani

Begin With Clean Nails

Before starting on your manicure and pedicure, be sure your toe and finger nails are free from polish using a remover that is free from acetone. Next, use a file or clippers to shape your nails gently into the best shape and length. Next, smooth your nails' surface using a buffer, and this will also help remove any unsightly yellow stains.

Soak & Scrub

Soak your hands for 2-3 minutes and your feet for 5 minutes. Now, you want to exfoliate. You can make an easy exfoliator by mixing a tablespoon each of sugar and baby oil gel. Then gently scrub away dry, dead cells. It will smell great and leave your skin feeling really soft. Rinse off your hands and feet and pat them dry.

Take Care of your Cuticles

Make your cuticles soft by rubbing some coconut or baby oil into them. Now your cuticles ought to be soft, so push them back using your orangewood stick for a nice shape. You also can use the tool for cleaning dirt that's beneath your nails. Now you want to massage your hands and feet. Get a moisturizer that is full of vitamins and put it onto your hands and feet. Pay close attention to your cuticles and heels. Before you go on to the next step, swipe your nail beds using your non-acetone remover to remove any moisturizer and oil.

Don't forget the base coat
Put on your base coat so that any ridges are smoothed and there's a surface that's even for the colour. You only need one coat.

Put your polish on
Put two layers of polish on your nails, letting your polish completely dry in between each of the coats. To make it look professional, swipe your polish down your nail's centre and on either side. You want to make your polish layers thin, since it will make the polish last longer and make the polish dry faster.

Shine it up
Putting your top coat on is going to add shine but it will also smooth away flaws and flubs. You only need one coat. To refresh your manicure or pedicure quickly during the week, put another top coat layer. It will make a big difference.

Relax
Simply chill and don't do anything while your nails are drying. Watch a movie, listen to some music, just don't do anything when you are letting them dry. Otherwise you are going mess up your manicure and pedicure.

Food Tips For Gorgeous Nails

Your nails are made of keratin which is a protein so this is why a protein-rich diet is important for great nail health. If you are vegetarian make sure your diet consists of foods like quinoa, beans, and meat substitutes like tofu and seitan. This will make sure you have a balanced diet and the nutrients you need for strong nails.

Following are some more foods which will keep your whole body healthy, but are especially good for beautiful nails.

Eggs

Eggs are full of protein, just ask anyone in the gym. The nail plate which is the hard see-through portion of your nail is made of protein. Eggs are also rich in B vitamins that are components of biotin, which will aid your nail growth.

Broccoli

So your body can properly use the protein you eat, it is essential to consume an amino acid called cysteine, which is found in the awesome vegetable broccoli. This mega veggie is also loads with some great vitamins.

Salmon

Why do our Norwegian friends have great nails? Well, their secret is eating plenty of salmon. This delicious fish has lots of protein and contains zinc, which helps your body absorb the protein you consume. Salmon also contains selenium and copper, which aid in the production of collagen which can help your nail growth.

Coconut Oil

If you eat healthy fats like coconut oil your body will be better at absorbing nutrients. Coconut oil also contains vitamins A, D, E, and K, to further strengthen your beautiful nails.

Chicken

Chicken also contains lots of vitamin B, zinc and protein which all help your nails grow strong.

Spinach

Spinach is just great for Popeye. This dark green veggie has vitamin E, iron, B vitamins, folate, and vitamin A, which all help nail strength and growth.

Brazil Nuts

These nuts are loaded with collagen-building selenium, zinc, vitamin B, and vitamin E. Snack on some of these for supermodel quality nails.

Skin Tips

One of the things that people will notice about you is your skin. Your skin is much different from how it will be when you are an adult. Remember that your skin is much more permeable, which means substances are more able to go into it than when you are an adult. This means you are going to have problems with irritation more than adults will. But you have the advantage that your skin will heal quicker.

Here are some skin tips that you can use:

1. Choose a scrub that you can use all over your body to get rid of your dead skin. Make sure that areas such as your chest, back, and shoulders are covered. If you have oily skin, gently scrub your T-zone so that you can get rid of and prevent blackhead problems.
2. Shave after your shower or bath. If you would rather wax, take a quick cold shower.
3. Always get enough sleep so that you can avoid dark circles and acne.
4. Always avoid smoking or being in smoky areas, especially confined spaces like in a car which can really damage your skin's appearance, as well as your lungs.

Lip Care:

You might be wondering why there's a separate section for lip care. That's because your lips' skin is much more sensitive than the skin on the other parts of your body. The reason for this is because it doesn't have the glands it needs for nourishing itself and your lips' skin is much more sensitive right now. It dries, bleeds, and cracks much more easily.

Here are a few things that you can do to keep your lips' skin supple and soft.

1. Exfoliate the skin on your lips, but use things like honey and sugar. Don't use a tooth brush even if its bristles are really soft.

2. Moisturize your lips frequently. Don't allow them to dry out.
3. Don't lick them and especially do not peel or pull off dry skin. These both cause a lot of damage which will take time to heal.
4. If your lips are chapped, don't put on lipstick. Lipstick will only highlight the chapped lips and make your lips drier.

5. Always look for expiration dates. Products that have expired contain less nutrients and possibly more bacteria and this can lead to problems with your skin.

Hair

If you are like a lot of teens, one of the most important things to you is your hair and how it looks. We know how you want your hair to look great and how you are looking for some really professional tips to make it look great.

To get you started, here are some tips that are going to make it simpler to have beautiful hair.
1. Be very careful when it comes to blonde highlights. You should stick closer to your hair's natural tones.
2. Get haircuts that are easy for you to manage such as layers. Layers will often save time when you are getting dressed since they look good with just about every type of hair.

3. If you have a problem with an oily scalp, save your money and reach for baby powder. Using baby powder at your roots will work wonders if you have light coloured hair. If your hair is dark, though, use a shampoo that's especially formulated for dry hair.

4. If you're looking for a style that is amazing, you shouldn't go overboard. There are plenty of styles that look great and hardly take any time. Put some loose curls into your hair using your barrel iron. Not only is it fast but it also helps with minimizing heat damage.

5. Sometimes it can seem like your hair is working against you and sometimes it works beautifully. What you need to know is that you need to care for it properly to get the best results. Whether you are styling it every day or you're just putting it into a fun ponytail, here are some useful tips to care for your hair to prevent those bad hair days.

Make sure it's clean

It's important that you start with a base of shiny and clean hair. Wash it regularly, which can mean a few times each week or even every day. The shampoo will clean your hair and scalp by removing oil, product build-up, and dirt, but this can also remove your hair's natural oils which help your hair be bouncy, controllable, and shiny. You should choose a shampoo that's specifically made for your hair type. Whether you have straight, flat, stressed out, coloured, frizzy, or curly hair, there's a type of shampoo for you. If you are always swimming, you can find a shampoo that is made for you too. Follow the product instructions and understand when it's time to wash your hair.

How you should shampoo your hair

Soak your hair with water. Then apply the shampoo made for your type of hair. Only use the amount of shampoo so that you're working up a great lather and rinse your hair well.

Moisturize

Conditioner can be used for putting moisture in your hair so it is easier for you to brush or comb and tangle free. Read the conditioners' descriptions before buying them and find the one that will fit the needs of your hair. Follow the product directions and use the correct amount for your hair's length.

How You Should Condition

After you have shampooed your hair, rinse it well and then squeeze the excess water out of your hair. Put the right amount of conditioner in your hand. Then rub your palms together so that it's on both of your hands. Start at your hair's ends and then go upward to apply your conditioner. For the best results, read and follow the product's directions, which include the length of time that you should leave your conditioner in the hair. Rinse using lukewarm or cool water until your hair is no longer slimy from the product.

Go Curly

For those of you with hair that is naturally curly, use it to your advantage. After you have washed your hair, don't use a towel to dry it. It's going to break up your curls and cause it to be frizzy. Rather, gently scrunch it in your towel to remove any excess water. Use products that you enjoy and then allow your hair to naturally dry. If you really want to use your dryer, use an attachment known as a diffuser. Dry it with your head bent over, using your fingers to scrunch your hair.

If your hair is straight and you want some curls, using your towel, blot the excess water from your hair gently. Add some mousse or gel. Then twist small amounts of your hair into small ringlets. Hold these ringlets in place using some bobby pins or you can wrap these sections in some cushioned rollers. Use your hair dryer or sleep that way overnight. When your hair is totally dry, spray it using a lightweight spray. Remove the pins and curlers and then shake your hair out. Use your fingers to comb your hair. Do this a few different times, using sections that are different sizes to make your curls so that you can see what will work best for you.

Go Straight

Are you a girl who has slightly curly or naturally wavy hair? Maybe you want a change and you want to try straight hair. First, squeeze out your excess water. Then, put something on your hair to protect it from the heat. Put an attachment on your hair dryer so that you can concentrate the heat on a single section. Divide up your hair into eight different sections and then dry a single section.

Pull your hair straight gently using your brush while drying it so that you have an even, smooth finish. If you're aiming for a finish that is extra smooth, you can smooth out the frizzy pieces with a flat iron.

If your hair's really curly and you want straight hair, you can use the tips that are above or you might also need to use a straightener or relaxer. Speak to your parents beforehand to make sure they approve and to find out if they can give you any recommendations. They might make an appointment at a salon where someone can help you with keeping your hair straight longer.

Be Healthy & Protect Your Beautiful Hair

Hair's a reflection of how healthy you are. If you're eating a diet that is well-balanced, getting plenty of sleep, and exercising, your hair's going to show it. When you aren't in good health, your hair isn't going to be in good health either.

To care for your hair, it's also important to be very gentle so that you are protecting it. You shouldn't use water that is too cold or too hot. You should also protect it from the damage of heat when you are using things like blow dryers to flat irons or curling irons. These are the things that can affect your hair and make it dry. It's best to use a moisturizing conditioner and shampoo to help reduce the amount of damage your hair will have from styling. Also think about the environment – wear a scarf, cap, or hat if you're able to so that you can protect your hair from being over-exposed to salt, chlorinated water, the sun, air pollution, and wind.

When you use these tips to care for your hair, you're going to learn how you can keep your hair strong and healthy, and you'll have some great hair that looks wonderful and is easy to work with.

Makeup Tips

Now we have arrived at the section that you have probably been waiting for: all about make-up with some very useful make-up tips.

The Ancient Egyptians, both men and women, were wearing distinct make up from as early as 4,000BC. It wasn't just the men and women of Egypt either. The statues of their gods and goddesses were adorned with different types of cosmetics. The higher the status of the person the more make-up they wore. Japanese women began using powder on their faces made from rice centuries ago. At about the same time French women used chalk-based powders on their faces while Greek women used red iron to decorate their lips.

Every woman is beautiful, special, and unique and has something defining about her which one day a man will fall in love with. Yet, not enough women feel confident about themselves, especially during their teen years.

As teenagers, many girls already start applying make-up to go to school looking as grownup as they can. They ask their mums if they can wear blusher and mascara, so they can be popular and perhaps get the attention of the boys.

Some girls just love dressing up and putting on make-up, others to impress. One long-time friend confessed to me once that she thought she had awful bags under her eyes. In fact she said she felt like this since she was about 12. Then she discovered the power of concealer and was truly thankful. I also read recently that the average woman spends a cool $15,000 total during her lifetime on make-up, with $3,770 of that going toward mascara alone!

So, let's jump straight in to some make-tips from the experts which I am sure you are going to find very useful.

General Makeup Tips

- Don't buy anything without testing it first. Ask for some samples to be sure it won't make you break out.
- Don't pair smoky eyes and dark lips, since it often looks tacky on young faces.
- Use your very best features to your advantage. If your eyes are pretty, lining them will get them more attention. If your lips are awesome, use flattering lipstick or gloss to get them some attention.
- Don't use foundation if you have acne. If you do, find a formula that's free of oil.
- Pat your concealer on using your fingers instead of rubbing it on.
- Put your sunscreen on before your makeup or use makeup that has sunscreen in it.

5 Eyeliner Mistakes to Avoid

Putting too much on your bottom lid

When you put too much on your bottom lid, especially when you use a colour that is really dark, it can cause your eyes to look smaller. Plus, you will have a higher chance of smudges under your eyes. If you really want to give your lower lid definition, use a taupe or light brown eye shadow or a light coloured pencil.

Not putting it on evenly

It's really frustrating when you need to wipe off a line on your top lid using makeup remover over and over before getting it right. To keep your liner straight, don't tug at your eyes' outer corners. This may cause your skin to become crinkled and as a result you won't have a smooth line. Try looking down and pointing up with your chin, so that your lids are partially closed but they're still seeable. If you're using a gel liner, apply it using your slanted brush for a look that's smoother. It's also possible to use a light coloured pencil to draw your line so you have a guide.

Only sticking to brown and black

Some nude or white liner on your lower eyelid can do a lot to help you with looking refreshed and awake. Pull gently upon your under-eye, then trace that line between your inside rim and lower lashes.

Not knowing what gel, pencil, and liquids are

The pencil eyeliner works best when you don't have a lot of time. They are quick to use and they don't smear. Gel eyeliners are for a more glamorous look, they're water-resistant, and they give you more control about the thickness. Liquid eyeliners are the more advanced type. They are more precise when they are applied, but they also require a really steady hand when you're using them. They are not good for when you are first starting out.

Not smudge-proofing

You are able to do this easily. Apply the eyeliner using a small brush or pencil, and then trace this line using a powder shadow which matches. So that it will last longer, wet the shadow brush using Visine.

Eye Shadow

Did you know that all eye shadow colours are not created equal? Some of them are going to look better than others based on your eye colour and your skin tone. So here is some information about choosing the right eye shadow colour for you.

Brown Eyes

If your eyes are brown, you are truly blessed because you have the widest range of colours that will look good on your eyes. So if your eyes are like Megan Fox, Rachel Bilson or Kate Bosworth here are the colours that you can wear and look wonderful.

Best eye shadow shades for brown eyes
- Neutral colours like dark brown and grey
- Grey, beige, bronze are great for a smoky look
- Blue, particularly turquoise or crystal blue
- Purple
- Copper
- Silver /Coral
- Gold
- Aqua
- Mahogany
- Blunt orange
- Amber

Hazel Eyes

If you were born with hazel eyes, there are colours that look best for your eye colour. Wearing these eye colours is going to help you with accentuating your eyes and making them more beautiful. If your eyes are similar to Marisa Miller, Petra Nemcova or Sofia Vergara here we go.

Best eye shadow colours for eyes that are hazel
- Purple, particularly dark purple, lavender, plum, eggplant, and others for accentuating your eyes' green hues.
- Neutral / Gold, bronze, and yellow / Brown
- Green, particularly emerald and olive

Blue Eyes

If you have beautiful blue eyes there are some colours that are going to help you with looking great. So if your eyes are like Gotham starlet Makenzie Leigh or Olivia Rose Keegan let's go.

Best Eye shadow colours for Blue Eyes
- Dark brown / Orange
- Cool colours like violet, pale blue, dark blue, midnight blue, turquoise, and pale pink.

- Neutral colours like grey, camel, khaki, chocolate brown, and white.

Green Eyes

Do you have beautiful green eyes? If so, maybe you are wondering if there's a certain colour of eye shadow that you should be wearing. Just follow the lead of Amber Skye, gorgeous Virginia Kiss or even German starlet Bianca Schumacher with these colours.

Best eye shadow colours for eyes that are green

- Cream, coral, khaki, copper, mauve,
- Mocha, caramel, mocha, copper.
- Neutral colours particularly grey
- Beige
- Tan
- Gold
- Plum
- Peach
- Violet
- Green
- Charcoal

Now that we have gone over the colours based on the colour of your eyes, we are going to go over some of the colours based on your skin tone.

Eye Shadow Based on Skin Colour – Olive, Brown, Medium, Black

You skin colour has a big influence of the eye shadow colours you go for. Generally, the colour of your skin will be one of the following:

Eye shadows for Different Skin Colours

- Black (this will range from being very dark brown to being black)

- Brown (this is dark brown) / Olive (this is moderate brown)
- Medium (this is white to a medium brown)
- Fair (white) / Light (very pale white)

The information below is based on fair and dark skin colours and then we will mention cool and warm undertones. Here are some tips for choosing your eye shadow colours based on your skin tones.

Eye Shadow Colours if You Have Fair Skin

If you have fair skin, you shouldn't use dark grey eye shadow colours. This could create a beautiful smoky look, but if you have pale skin you may end up looking bruised.

Use cool pink, golds, purples, soft greens, light brown, and medium grey. In other words, go for light coloured earth tones. If you wear dark shades they may overpower your eyes. When it comes to contours, select colours that are a couple shades darker compared with your skin. This is going to ensure that the colour isn't overwhelming your eyes.

If you have dark skin, it's important to select vibrant colours since they are going to be toned down when they are applied to your eyes. If you select softer shades, they're going to fade away because of the colour of your skin. Your eye shadow needs to be deep in pigmentation. Colours such as metallic golds and purples are great.

Eye Shadow Colours for Girls with Dark Skin

If you have warm skin tones, you should choose light brown, pink, light brown, bronze, coral, and soft green. If you have a cool skin tone, you should choose lilac, teal, dark green, grey, turquoise, and silver.

Eye Shadow Colours for Various Hair Colours

The colour of your hair is essential when you are choosing your eye shadow. Here are some colours that you should choose based on the colour of your hair.

- Brown and Black hair - Eye shadow colours if you have brown or black hair include purple, green, yellow, black and brown. Neutrals like beige and gold will also work well. If you have brown hair, you can use just about any colour without an issue and they will look great.
- Blonde - Usually if you are blonde your skin is fair. The colours for eye shadow that you should use are grey, black, green, gold, and pink.
- Red - If you have red hair, you can wear pink, olive, gold, and black since they will work well with your intense hair colour.

Lipstick

If you are looking for a colour of lipstick that is going to work best for you, one of the things that you want to do is to consider your skin's tone. There are colours that look better with certain tones than others. Below is your guide to finding the right lipstick based on your skin tone.

Light Skin Tones
- What will look best - If you have lighter skin, you will do best with wearing berry and wine reds that have blue undertones, deep plum-reds, beige and brown lipsticks that have pink undertones, and pinks that have blue undertones. If your undertones are warm, you will look great in colours like browns with slightly bronze or golden shimmers to them, caramels, or cappuccino.
- What you should avoid - If your undertones are cool and pink, stay away from orange-reds, light browns that have

yellow undertones, plus any kinds of shades that could overpower your light complexion such as really hot pinks.

Light Olive/Medium Skin tones

What will look best - If your skin tone is light olive or medium, you should choose blue-reds, brownish reds, medium brown having pink or yellow undertones, coffee browns, and deep reds.

Olive Skin Tones

What will look best - Deeper red and brown shades and dark berry colours

What you should avoid – Pale pinks, pink-reds, orange-reds, and mauves

Medium-Brown Skin Tones

What will look best - Berry pinks, medium plums having yellow undertones, berry pinks, and brown reds

What you should avoid - Pinks that are too light or cool, orange, pastel shades

Dark Skin Tones

What will look best - You can wear deep, dark shades, reds that have blue undertones, reddish browns such as deep plums, raisin, coffee brown, deep rose, and mahogany

What you should avoid - Pastel shades, pinks, or orange

Trial and Error

Finding the perfect shade of lipstick often takes some time. One of the best methods is to take a tester and then swipe the colour onto your fingertips. Your finger pads are going to be closer to your lip colour when compared with your hand, so this will give you an accurate idea of the way it is going to look when you are wearing it.

To get the best idea of how it will look is to test it on your lips. There are some companies which might have some miniature lipsticks that you can use for testing. The other option is to buy the cheap brands for experimenting with the colours before you buy one that is more expensive or that has a better formula.

Mascara

A lot of girls have misconceptions when they first start wearing mascara. One of the funniest and earliest episodes of the show Full House was when DJ and Kimmy were wearing mascara for the first time and they opened their mouths and eyes really wide in order to put mascara on. So here are 10 tips that you can use to correctly wear mascara.

Select the Right Colour
A lot of girls just go for black mascara. That's because it is subtly dramatic. It also flatters most skin tones. But it also often looks harsh on girls with really fair skin or looks really obvious on girls who want a more natural look. Brown's a great choice for girls who want a less-bold look.

Put On Some Eyeliner
If you have sparse or fair eyelashes, you might not think the mascara is going to be enough. It can also be hard for many girls to put mascara on to their eyelashes' base. Draw an eyeliner line along your eyelid, getting as close as you can to your eyelash line. If you can, select a colour that's very close to your mascara colour. This will help with blending in. This line is going to make your eyelashes look thicker. It's also going to let you make the illusion that you have full mascara coverage even if you aren't able to completely cover your lashes.

Wiggle Your Applicator Brush
For a coat of mascara that is more even and gives you better coverage, begin with your brush at your lashes' base like you usually do. However, when you draw your brush over your lashes, wiggle your brush from one side to another. This is going to coat your

lashes' sides as well as their bottoms, meaning you will get more volume. Also, it will make sure that there's even coverage on every lash. This can take some practice to get it down, but it will also help you apply your mascara quicker.

Apply More Than One Light Coat
Even though wiggling your brush is going to help you with getting better coverage over your lashes, you shouldn't count on a single swipe. Many girls find that putting on more than one coat is best. You can go for the single or double coat look for school and you can make it more dramatic for an evening out or a date. Give it some time and allow it to layer. Make sure that you apply coats before your first coat has dried completely, otherwise you are going to get clumps.

Get a Comb for Your Eyelashes
If you are still having problems with clumps, eyelash combs can be a big help. They are made to even out your lashes and remove clumps. Apply your mascara and then, while it's wet, run your comb from your eyelashes' base and up. You can buy an actual brush or you can also use a clean wand. If you keep a wand on hand for this, regularly wash it so that you don't have problems with bacteria growth. You can also apply your mascara, wipe your brush off using a tissue, and then use it for combing your lashes.

Use a Curler Before Your First Coat
You can shape your eyelashes using an eyelash curler. The curler positions your lashes to better frame your eyes and it also brightens your eyes because it moves your eyelashes out of the way. A mascara that's designed to curl your lashes will be a good choice if you're not comfortable using the curler. It is going to work a lot better and give you results that are more consistent. Just use on the corner near your eyelashes' roots and press down for approximately 30 seconds. Don't try curling your lashes after you put the mascara on since mascara often sticks to your curler and pulls your lashes out.

Once your lashes have been curled to your satisfaction, put your mascara on.

Get the Brush that's Right for You

There are a lot of different sizes and shapes of brushes so you want to find one that is best for your needs. Some girls want curved brushes made to reach all of their lashes at one time and some prefer straight brushes. One way to maximize the brush control is to bending the brush's end at an angle that's 90 degrees to your wand. This makes it a lot easier and more natural for application.

Put the Mascara on Clean Eyelashes

A lot of girls find it's easy to transition their look from school to a date simply by putting on a couple of more coats. But the greatest results come from starting over. The old mascara may flake off and add some clumps and bumps to your eyelashes. This can even irritate your eyes. Old mascara's also more brittle, which means your eyelashes might not be in the right position and shape. Think about buying a remover for eye makeup. The best one will remove your eye makeup, reduce eye irritation and infection risk, and regular use will give you healthier, better-looking eyelashes.

Care for Your Mascara

When your mascara's in its best condition, it will glide onto your lashes much more smoothly and it will be healthier. Even though you may want to dunk your brush repeatedly into the tube so that you are able to get a lot of product on your applicator, this can cause your mascara to dry out quicker. It's also essential to replace your mascara monthly, even if you have leftover product. Bacteria grow in the mascara, and keeping your tube fresh will make it much safer for you to use. Fresh mascara will also be a lot easier to use since it won't be old enough to dry out.

Give Your Lashes Drying Time

Once you have applied your mascara, it may be tempting for you to apply your other makeup. But most girls, particularly those who have long lashes, should wait a couple of seconds to be sure the mascara's dry completely. There are times when even blinking is going to make the mascara rub off on the area beneath your eyes, leading to smudges and dark spots. Have patience and try waiting before you move your eyelids or blink too much.

Chapter 4
Teen Health & Your Body

As this is such a massive area, it deserves a full book on the topic of your health. However, I wanted to at least cover a few very important areas in this book which I feel are not talked about enough. You might find it difficult to get decent information on.

Please see *OMG I Feel Fat - A Teenagers' Guide to Health & Fitness* and other books in the **OMG Teen Book Series**, www.omgteenbookseries.com for more detailed information on Teen Health.

Essential Information about Acne

As a teenager, you are noticing that your body is going through a lot of changes. Some of these changes are fun, some of them are unpleasant. One of the things that you may notice happening to you are these spots on your skin that may make you say Ewww! Sometimes they happen right in the middle of your nose! And the worst is when they show up on the worst possible day, like when it is class picture day or when you are going to a dance.

Unfortunately, those spots, also known as zits or pimples, are part of growing up. Lots of teens get them. Your friends might give you some tips on how you can get rid of your zits. But a lot of the information that you get from your friends, unless they have a doctor for a parent, is likely to be wrong. So let's look at the myths and professional facts about pimples and acne.

Myth 1: I can clear my skin up by getting a tan
Fact: Even though a tan might help to mask your acne, sun can make your skin very irritated and dry, which can result in more breakouts down the road. There's no proven link between preventing acne and sun exposure. The truth is that you have to be careful about too much

sun exposure, since it can cause skin cancer and premature aging. You want to look young and beautiful as long as possible right? It's best to use sunscreen of at least SPF 15 with the word nonacnegenic or noncomedogenic on its label. This means the sunscreen isn't going to clog your pores, which is very important.

Myth 2: If I wash my face a lot, I will have fewer breakouts

Fact: Even though washing will help remove oil and dirt from pores, you can actually make your acne worse when you wash your face excessively. Excessive washing leads to irritation and dryness in your skin, which can lead to more breakouts. You also should avoid scrubbing your skin. The best way to wash your face is with water and mild soap, washing it in gentle circular motions and then gently patting your face dry when you are done. You should do this once in the morning, then again at night before bed. In addition, if you exercise, you should wash your face after exercising.

Myth 3: If I pop my pimples, they will go away quicker

Fact: Although popping your pimples may seem like a good way to make it less noticeable for that dance, it also will encourage it to be there longer. When you are squeezing your zits and pimples, you're actually pushing all that dangerous stuff like bacteria, oil, and dead cells further into your skin. This leads to more redness and swelling. This can also cause a brown or red mark, or even a scar. Sometimes these marks can stay around for a while. The true scars, which are pits and dents, last forever. Not really worth popping the pimple to look good temporarily, right?

Myth 4: I shouldn't wear makeup because I want my skin to be clear

Fact: You can wear makeup if you choose cosmetics that say non-comedogenic or nonacnegenic. The truth is some of the concealers have salicylic acid or benzoyl peroxide in them which can help with fighting acne. You also can try using benzoyl peroxide creams which are tinted so they can help hide your pimples while they're helping with treating them.

If you've had problems with moderate or severe acne, it's a good idea to speak with your dermatologist to find out what cosmetics you should use. In some cases they might suggest that you shouldn't use makeup or you should only use certain brands.

Myth 5: I shouldn't eat certain foods because they cause acne
Fact: This is one of the things that most teens believe about acne.
Your friends might have told you that eating hamburgers or chocolate can cause acne, but these are just myths. The truth is that food has little to do with breakouts. The thing that causes your acne is the same thing that is causing all the changes in your body – hormones. This is why so many of your friends have spots right now. Those hormones that are causing your breasts to grow and your period to start are the same ones that cause your glands to produce more oil. This oil can clog up your pores and lead to acne. Latest research has not shown a connection between particular foods and skin health. So while those foods might not affect the condition of your skin, they will affect your overall health.

Myth 6: If I keep on getting breakouts, I should use a lot more acne medication to make them stop.
Fact: Since acne medicine has agents to dry up your skin like salicylic acid and benzoyl peroxide, using a lot of it can actually make things worse. It will make your skin dry and irritated and it can cause more blemishes.
So, now that you know the facts about acne, let's see what you can do about those annoying pimples. Here are some tips based on information from the WebMD website.

Start Out Using OTC Acne Treatments

When you are looking for over the counter treatments, you should look for ones that say they contain salicylic acid and benzoyl peroxide. According to Charles E. Crutchfield III, MD, who is a professor of dermatology at the University of Minnesota Medical School, "Products that contain salicylic acid unplug the pores and those with benzoyl peroxide are mild anti-inflammatories and also kill or stop bacteria from growing." The one thing to keep in mind is that if you are a person of colour, it may not be a good idea to use benzoyl peroxide since it may decolourize your skin. It is best to use it under the supervision of a dermatologist.

Don't overdo. According dermatologists, using a lot of acne products could make your skin worse. Stay clear of the skincare products that have alcohol in them, since this can cause your skin to become irritated and cause outbreaks.

Care for Your Face Daily

Here's a three minute routine that dermatologists recommend will help improve your skin quality.
Wash your hands first: You MUST always wash your hands thoroughly before you wash your face. Doctors advise us that we should wash our hands for at least 20 seconds after using the toilet to make sure our hands are bacteria free. This is one of the benefits of using a bidet sprayer rather than toilet paper, as your hands are exposed to much less bacteria when you use a bidet sprayer.

1. **Wash your face gently two times per day**
    Use the tips of your fingers rather than a washcloth and some lukewarm water. Use a mild non-soap cleanser for one wash and then a wash made with 2 ½% benzoyl peroxide the second time.
2. **Perform spot treatments**
    Dot your problem areas using a product made with 2% salicylic acid after you've washed your face using a cleanser. Don't do this step when you have done the wash with benzoyl peroxide.
3. **Use Moisturizer**
    After you have cleaned your face, use a moisturizer that says *non-comedogenic, nonacnegenic*, or *oil free*. During the daytime, use one that has at least an SPF of 15.

It's also very important to wash your hair daily if you have oily hair and don't use oily gels. You want to keep any kind of oil off your face. In addition, be careful when you are playing sports. You should wash your face after you exercise. Anything which holds sweat upon your skin, such as a helmet or baseball cap can make your acne worse. So wipe down your helmet straps using alcohol before and after you have finished playing. If you discover pimples in other areas, like your back or chest, remove sweaty clothes following sports and take a shower. If you have pimples in other areas, use a mild cleanser on those areas or 2½% benzoyl peroxide.

How to Solve Emergency Pimple Problems

Sometimes, no matter how well you take care of your skin, you wake up to find a huge pimple on a very important day. When this happens, here is some advice which should help.

- Use a warm compress such as a warm wet washcloth and keep it there for 10 minutes. This will help your zit get a head on it.
- Try using spot treatments with a product that has 2% salicylic acid. Apply even, gentle pressure to the zit using two Q-tips. If anything's ready to exit your zit, this is when it will happen. Do not squeeze and never do it with your fingers.
- If it's not draining, grab some ice and use it on the pimple to reduce swelling.
- Dr. Wechsler also says that you can use some 1% hydrocortisone cream in emergencies, but she doesn't recommend using it constantly for acne problems.

For hiding and spot treating pimples, use blemish eraser sticks with salicylic acid on one of its ends and makeup on its other.

What Dermatologists Can Do To Help You

If you still aren't happy with your spots, make an appointment with a dermatologist. They will be able to prescribe stronger medicine for acne. They can also use heat and laser treatments to get rid of the bacteria that are on your skin, along with corticosteroid injections for easing large, painful acne lesions.

If your acne has already caused scars, a dermatologist can use things such as dermabrasion, surgery, chemical peels, skin fillers, and laser resurfacing to decrease them.

Acne Advice for People of Colour

If you have darker skin, you might have to deal with different problems related to acne than those with lighter skin. These problems are:

Dark spots - These are spots that appear in the areas in which blemishes healed. These will generally disappear as time goes by. But it's also helpful to use products that lighten your skin. If you have a dermatologist, he or she might also suggest using concealer makeup to cover these spots to make them less noticeable.

Keloids - Keloids are raised scars which are bigger than your original blemish and can be difficult to remove. You shouldn't let acne go for a long time without treating it so that keloids can be prevented.

Good Advice for All Teens

Beware of falling for miracle cures. Unfortunately, there aren't any overnight cures that can get rid of acne yet. If you hear of someone online or on the television who promises a guaranteed, fast acne treatment, you will be wasting your money.

You have to use your acne treatment regularly and commit to using it for at least two months before you are going to see any type of results. Then you can decide if it is for you or you want to try something else.

Even if a product is labeled noncomedogenic or nonacnegenic, it's important that you stop using it and speak with your doctor if you notice that it's causing breakouts or irritation.

If OTC acne medicine isn't working, you should speak with your dermatologist or doctor. In addition, if you're taking a prescription medication for acne, be sure that you're following the instructions that your doctor gives you – some of the medicines can take as long as two months before making big difference.

All About Constipation

It is often very difficult for teens to talk about anything to do with the bathroom, even with their best friend or their parents. Therefore, this chapter is for you, so you can get the information you need, but are perhaps not comfortable asking anyone about.

It's very common for anyone to have a problem with pooping at one time or another. So you should not have to put up with constipation just because you don't know how to deal with it. Relax because it's usually not a big problem. Let the following advice lead you to a better quality of life by learning about some common problems with constipation, and some handy solutions.

What is Constipation?

If you are constipated it only means that you are having trouble pooping, often called a bowel movement, or what your friend might call "having a no.2, dropping a log" or any number of terms. When you are constipated it usually means your poop is too hard and you may strain when they try to go to the toilet. You could be constipated if you are going to the toilet less than 3 or 4 times per week. Often people may wait so long to go to the toilet that they get even more constipated. Medically, constipation is defined as fewer than three stools per week and severe constipation as less than one stool per week.

Why am I Constipated?

There are some medical situations which can cause constipation, like irritable bowel syndrome, diabetes, low thyroid, and pregnancy. If you have to take strong medicine, this could also cause constipation. Not having enough water, a disruption in your regular routine, like when you are traveling, eating large amounts of dairy products or even stress can cause constipation. Often though, constipation happens because you do not have enough fibre in your diet or you have been waiting too long to go to the bathroom.
The good news is that dietary and lifestyle changes can keep you "regular" and help you feel better.

How Do I Know I Have Constipation?

There is no perfect number for the amount of times you should be pooping per day, but you will generally feel better if you are going every day or at least every other day.

Not going to the toilet can give you a stomach ache. Some people with constipation may notice bright red blood when they are going to the toilet. This bleeding is a sign that the anus has been irritated.
This can cause an anal fissure which is a tear in your anus or a haemorrhoid, which is swollen tissue near the anus. A haemorrhoid is often painful and often bleeds when you go to the toilet. If this happens, it can be scary to see blood, but the soreness and bleeding will generally go away when you start having regular and softer poops again.

It is always a good idea to arrange an appointment with your G.P or family doctor so she can tell you what help you need. Better safe than sorry as they say. Your G.P will probably ask about your diet to examine if you are eating enough fibre. She'll also want to know how much water you are drinking each day.

Some Useful Constipation Tips

As a teenager you always have so much to do, such as with school, your sports schedule, your hobbies and other outside of school activities. Maybe you don't have much privacy, or perhaps even finding a bathroom can be challenging. But if you have been uncomfortable because of constipation, it is time to think about how you can feel better!

You will probably want to plan ahead by knowing where the bathrooms are, whether you are at school, playing sports, or hanging out in other places. Finally, you'll need to slowly add more fibre to your diet and drink more water.

Some Useful Tips:

Here are some really useful actionable tips which will help you rid yourself of constipation.

- Please make sure you drink plenty of water, at least 8 to 10 big glasses per day.
- Get up early enough to do some light exercises in your bedroom. Then have breakfast, leaving enough time before you shower. It is your aim to have a toilet visit before you leave for school.
- Make sure you are doing some regular exercise every day even if it is only going for a walk.
- Start a habit of going to the bathroom at the same time every day. Try 15 to 20 minutes after your meal. You can usually get into a routine if you eat your meals around the same time every day.

- Don't force the pace when you get to a bathroom. Take a magazine and relax. If you are relaxed, you should find it easier to go.
- Make sure you are getting enough fibre in your diet

Some High Fibre Healthy Eating Tips

Yes! There are foods that tend to cause constipation and there are foods that tend to help your digestive system process food and help get rid of the waste. Foods containing fibre can help prevent constipation. Fibre is found in fruits, vegetables, whole grains, beans, legumes, and nuts.

Here are some healthy eating tips to increase your fibre intake:

A Healthy Breakfast:

- Pure olive oil can help to relieve constipation. It stimulates your digestive system, which helps get things moving through your colon, and taken regularly it can prevent constipation as well. Consume one tablespoon of olive oil on an empty stomach for best results.
- Eat a high-fibre cereal like All-Bran or a bowl of oatmeal.
- Coffee can do more than perk you up. Caffeine is a natural stimulant for the digestive system, so can stimulate your bowels. Try a cup in the morning to help get you up and running. If you are not much of a coffee fan, try half a cup to start with.
- Try a fruit smoothie for breakfast, like cutting up a few different fruits, toss some berries in and a slice of melon or apricots.
- Have a small glass of prune juice.

A Healthy Lunch:

- Have minestrone or lentil soup.
- Make your sandwiches with whole grain bread, and eat the crusts.
- Add some veggies to your sandwich, like tomato, avocado, or cucumber.
- Have some plums, pears, apples or nuts

A Healthy Dinner:

- Aloe is a great plant and so a good idea to get one. Pure aloe vera gel from the plant can soothe your tummy. It is more concentrated than commercial aloe juice so don't use more than 2 tablespoons. If you don't have an aloe plant, then you can drink aloe juice for similar results.
- You should have some vegetable with every meal. Try some broccoli, pumpkin, green beans, sprouts, carrots, or perhaps asparagus with your evening meal.
- Try a side portion of whole grain brown rice or whole wheat pasta.
- Be sure to drink lots of water when you increase your fibre intake. Otherwise your constipation may actually get worse! Also, increase your fibre intake slowly to prevent feeling bloated or having diarrhoea.

Are there any foods I should avoid if I'm constipated?

Some foods are high in fat and low in fibre, like cookies, ice cream and other sweet things. You should probably limit foods like cheese and other dairy products, processed foods, and meat. They may make your constipation worse. Try to choose higher fibre foods if you have problems with constipation.

What if I don't like high fibre foods?

I'm sure your parents tried to encourage you to eat healthy foods when you were younger. And perhaps they sometimes 'tried' too hard. If you feel you are not a believer in any high fibre foods like fruit and vegetables, perhaps I can suggest you give these foods another try. When I was younger I was not especially fond of apples. But knowing they were so good for me I tried slicing them up, and taking the core out. I found that eating the apple was much easier when I had the slices on a small plate while I was doing my homework or watching TV. Why don't you give this idea a try? Your hands don't become so sticky, plus it's much easier to eat smaller pieces than having to bite into a whole apple.

The same goes with drinking water. When I was an early teen I found out that drinking water was essential to a healthy life. However, I knew I didn't like it, so what could I do? I started by drinking a glass of water every time I washed my teeth, and gradually built up to over ten glasses every day. You'll be surprised, but you will probably come to love water, if you give it a real good try. Keep a jug of water in the fridge if you are able to drink tap water in your area. This ensures you have a glass of cool water anytime and prevents you wasting water when you have to run the tap.

What about taking laxatives?

I do not advise taking enemas or laxatives from the pharmacy. They are not natural and it is better to get your diet and exercise routines right, before thinking of taking these kinds of products.

When should I arrange an appointment with my family doctor?

It is a good idea to contact your family doctor if you have:
- Constipation that gets worse or doesn't get better
- Bloody stools, vomiting, or stomach pain
- A loss of appetite, a fever

It is common to be constipated once in a while, but if you have trouble or pain a lot of the time, or if you notice blood when you poop, you should make an appointment and talk to your family doctor. Decreasing foods that cause constipation, increasing fibre, drinking more water, and exercising will help keep you regular.

Your Own Super Computer – The Brain

The brain is the great invention ever, without question. For an idea of the complexity of the brain: a one millimetre cube of brain matter can contain between 35 and 70 million neurons, and a complete brain somewhere between 86 and 100 billion neurons. All together that makes the world's greatest super computer.

The brain is so advanced that we are always learning more about it. Interesting research currently going on is looking at how experience and environment affect the future abilities and behaviour of teens. In other words, to what extent does what a teen does and learns shape her brain over the rest of a lifetime. Furthermore, powerful new technologies have enabled experts to track the growth of the brain and to investigate the connections between brain function, development, and behaviour.

The latest research has also turned up some surprises, among them the discovery of striking changes taking place during the teen years. These findings have altered long-held assumptions about when the brain matures. Your brain is going through a lot of growth and development, and so right now your brain doesn't look like it will when you're in your early 20s.

The more we learn, the better we are able to understand the abilities and vulnerabilities of teens, and the significance of this stage in your life for life-long mental health.

Perhaps one of the most remarkable pieces of evidence in this latest research is the finding that different parts of the brain develop at different rates. The parts of the brain responsible for more "top-down" control, hallmarks of adult behaviour, such as controlling impulses and planning ahead, develop last.

Although the human brain represents only 2% of the body weight, it receives 15% of the cardiac output, 20% of total body oxygen consumption, so it is vital you feed your brain well.

Foods That Are Good For Your Brain Include:

1. **Blueberries** – are effective in improving or delaying short term memory loss.
2. **Avocados** - besides this creamy treat being rich in the anti-oxidant vitamin E, it contributes to healthy blood flow which means a healthy brain. Avocados also lower blood pressure which your brain will also love.
3. **Green tea** - is perhaps the healthiest beverage on the planet. It is loaded with antioxidants and nutrients that have powerful effects on the body, including improved brain function. The chemical properties of green tea promote the generation of brain cells, providing benefits for memory and learning.
4. **Fish oil** – is good for healthy brain function, the heart, joints and general wellbeing.
5. **Whole grains** - brain cannot work without energy. The ability to concentrate and focus comes from the adequate, steady supply of energy - in the form of glucose in our blood to the brain.
6. **Tomatoes** - evidence suggests a powerful antioxidant found in tomatoes, called lycopene, can help protect against free radical damage to cells.
7. **Broccoli** – is a great source of vitamin K, which is known to enhance cognitive function and improve brainpower.
8. **Sage** - has long had a reputation for improving memory.

9. **Pumpkin seeds** - daily amount of zinc is vital for enhancing memory and thinking skills.
10. **Vitamins** - B6, B12 and folic acid are known as the brain vitamins, and Vitamin C has long been thought to have the power to increase mental agility. Vitamin E is great for helping cognitive functions so that means plenty of nuts, leafy green vegetables, asparagus, olives, seeds, eggs, brown rice and whole grains.

Things That Are Bad For Your Brain Include:

1. **Refined foods** – if you eat too many of these foods (white flour, white sugar, white rice and soda) it can cause imbalances in your brain that cause you to feel irritable, distracted, tired or fidgety. To run at its best, your brain needs a steady supply of quality food throughout the day.
2. **Monosodium glutamate (MSG)** is a flavour enhancer often found in Chinese food, canned vegetables, soups and processed meats. While there is not definite evidence to link MSG with health problems, many researchers admit it could cause headaches, chest pain, and nausea for some people.
3. **Alcohol** - is a neurotoxin, which means it can poison your brain and kill your brain cells.

If you are interested in learning more about the brain, one of my favourite authors in this area is Dr. Daniel Amen who has written some excellent books about the brain.

The brain is obviously massively important for your health and general well-being, so look after it, and make sure you feed it the foods it needs.

Greg & Cristina Noland

Chapter 5
How To Beat Bullying

This chapter is all about bullying and what to do if you are bullied. This chapter will give you some actionable ideas how to manage social cruelty. Because having an effective plan will help you deal with social difficulties in an empowering way.

Unfortunately, bullying is a huge problem these days, and it is likely that you have faced bullying and friendship issues. Bullying often causes physical and psychological symptoms in victims like headaches, stomach aches, depression, and anxiety.

In the United States, school bullying statistics show that about one in four kids are bullied on a regular basis while experiencing some form of rejection by their classmates. Between cyber bullying and bullying at school, the school bullying statistics illustrate a huge problem with bullying and the American school system.

Professionals also say that in addition to causing mental health problems, bullying and social isolation can increase the likelihood a child will get poor grades, drop out of school, or develop substance abuse problems. It has become so bad that a lot of teens have actually committed suicide because they were bullied.

I can still remember to this day all about the time I was bullied by a gang when I was younger. But I did not let them win, and fought back by believing I was better than them. I would not allow them to defeat me. And you must not also. In fact years later I pity them because deep down I know they are most likely living very sad, pathetic lives.

Whether you have been unfortunate to be a victim of bullying or have had other difficult issues, every adult has been where you are

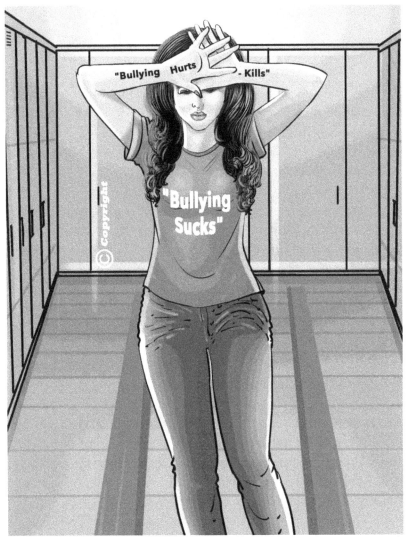

right now and we understand what you are going through. So sit back and please enjoy reading this book. We hope that you will find it very informative and that many of your questions will be answered. It is our mission through the information, advice and tips container in this book that it works as a resource to help you through your teenage years, and helps you realise that you are not alone. This Survival Guide for Teenage Girls will give you the strength to overcome some of the difficult problems you may have to face as a teenager.

Types of Bullying

First, let's look at the different kinds of bullying.

Physical Bullying:

Pushing, kicking, hitting someone, or even threatening that they will do it.

Ruining, hiding, or stealing another person's things.

Humiliation, hazing, and harassment – making another   person do things they don't want to.

Verbal Bullying:

Name calling / Taunting and teasing

Verbally abusing another person because of looks, what they are wearing, their possessions or their religion.

Relationship Bullying

Refusing to speak with someone

Excluding the person from activities or groups

Spreading rumours or lies about a person

Reasons Bullies Do It

Look powerful or tough

They are or were bullied

They want to be popular, show off, 'think' they are funny

They are jealous

To escape, deflect their own problems

If you are being bullied, research has shown that in some cases over 50% of children have been bullied, so you are not alone. Even though there are quite a few reasons why bullies have made you their target, the biggest reasons are usually your social standing or physical appearance.

Bullies often pick on the people that are different or who aren't fitting in. It might be due to the way you dress, hoe you act, or because you have a different race, sexual orientation or religion. It may simply be because you are new and you don't have any friends.

If You're Being Bullied, Here Are Some Things To Remember:
- **Do not blame yourself** – It's not your fault. It doesn't matter what another person does or says, you shouldn't be ashamed about how you feel or who you are.
- **Be proud of yourself** – No matter what bullies say, there are a lot of great things going for you. Remember that, rather than the messages the bullies are sending.
- **Always try to get some help** – Talk to an adult about what is going on, like a teacher, parent, or counsellor. Talking to a counsellor doesn't mean that you have done anything wrong.
- The bullying that you are currently facing will blow over. It will not last forever. Do not think it is never ending.
- **Learn how to cope with stress** – Finding ways to relieve stress can make you much more resilient so you don't feel overwhelmed by the bully. Meditation, exercise, talking positively to yourself, breathing exercises, and muscle relaxation are great ways to manage the stress that comes from being bullied.

Tips For Dealing With Bullies And Overcoming Being Bullied

There is no one solution to the problem of bullying and there is no one way for handling a bully. It can take experimenting with a few different responses before you are able to figure what is going to work best for you. To defeat a bully, you have to keep your self-control and self-sense.

Tip 1: Understand Bullying Truths

- **Walk away.** Bullies like knowing they've got control over you so you shouldn't react angrily or retaliate using physical force. If you're walking away, ignoring them, or assertively and calmly telling them you aren't interested in what they're saying, you're showing they're not controlling you.
- **Protect yourself.** in case you're not able to walk away and you're being hurt physically, do what you can to protect

yourself. Your first priority is your safety. You could take up a martial arts class as I did, and the bullying will stop once you learn the 'force'.

- **Report the bully to someone you trust**. If you do not report assaults and threats, bullies often become a lot more aggressive. Many times adults are able to find one or more ways to help the problem of the bully without telling the bully who told on them.

- **Repeat as it is necessary.** If the bully is relentless and you may have to be also. Report all of the bullying incidents until it is no longer happening. Remember, there's absolutely no reason that you should have to deal with bullying.

Tip 2: Reframe The Bullying Problem

Through changing your attitude towards the bully you will be able to get more control back.

- **Try to change your perspective**. A bully is a frustrated, unhappy person who is trying to control your feelings so that you feel bad, too. Don't allow them to have the satisfaction.

- **Examine the big picture**. Bullying is very common, but ask yourself what it means in the overall scheme of things. Is it going to matter next month, next year? Is it really worth being upset about? If your answer is no, put your energy and time elsewhere.

- **Remember the positive**. Think about the things that you love in life, including your gifts and positive qualities. Make up a list, put it on the wall next to your bed and look at it when you are feeling down.

- **Look for fun things**. If you are relaxed enough so that you are able to recognize how absurd a bully is and comment on it with some humour, you won't be the bully's target anymore.

- **Don't try controlling the uncontrollable**. A lot of things in life will be beyond your control, including how other people behave. Instead of stressing, focus on things you're able to control, like the way you react to the sad, pathetic bully.

- **Do not beat on yourself**. Do not make an incident of bullying a lot worse by replaying it or dwelling upon it. You should put your focus on all of the positive things in your life instead.
- **Use your Morning Ritual to boost your confidence (see Chapter 7)**. Always remember, if you think the bully is popular at school right now, they will not be later in life. More often than not they will be the ones who fail and have miserable lives.

Tip 3: Look For Support From Others Who Don't Bully

Having people that you trust and you are able to turn to for support and encouragement will boost your level of resilience when you are being bullied. Reach out and connect with real friends and family or look for ways to make new friends. There are a lot of people who are going to appreciate and love you for being you.

- **Find people who share your interests and values**. You might be able to make some friends at a book club, religious organization, or youth group. Join some kind of team, get a new hobby, get a part-time job or learn a sport.
- **Talk about your feelings**. Talk with a counsellor, coach, parent, or a friend you trust. Expressing what you are going through can often make an enormous difference in how you feel, even if the situation seems like it is not changing.
- **Give your confidence a boost**. Exercise is a wonderful way that you can make yourself feel good and it also helps with reducing stress. Take up a martial art like karate or kick box-ing or even just punch your pillow. It will help with working off anger.

How Do I Move On After Being Bullied?

Bullying is a traumatic event for just about anyone. Even after the bullying has stopped, you might be afraid, angry, anxious, or feel helpless. Your very first instinct might be withdrawal. But isolation is only going to make it worse. Connecting with others who didn't participate in the bullying is going to help you with healing. Do your best to maintain your healthy relationships and don't spend a lot of time alone.

- Give yourself some time to heal from the bullying trauma – Don't try forcing yourself to heal and prepare yourself for having volatile and difficult emotions. Let yourself feel what you're feeling without any guilt or judgment. Speak with someone that you trust so that you can get your feelings out.

- Overcome feeling helpless - You will be able to foster a feeling of control and hope by reaching out and helping others who are going through what you went through. Get active in anti-bullying campaigns in your school. You can also write notes to the people who helped you or you can volunteer in another way.

- Manage your anger in ways that are positive – Do not let your anger make you want to become a bully. Rather, find some healthy ways to manage your anger and learn the safe ways to cool down.

- Take good care of yourself – Make sure you're eating right, sleeping enough, and exercising. When your body is healthy, it allows you to cope with the stress and trauma that comes with being bullied.

Going Back To School After You Were Bullied

Going back to school and facing the bullies can be really frightening. It is estimated that 160,000 children miss school every day due to fear of attack or intimidation by other students. Source: National Education Association. At first, you may feel you want to change schools or not go to school altogether by getting home schooling. However, this can interrupt your education, cause you to become cut off from your friends, and limit future socializing opportunities. Unfortunately, there are bullies in every school, so going to a different school isn't a good option.

- Rather than putting your focus on the things and people you don't like about going to school focus on the aspects and people at school you like.

- Through reporting the bullying and getting the school involved, it may be possible to change some of your classes to put distance between the bullies and you. If it isn't possible, a teacher who is sympathetic may be able to give you a different seat.

- Find new activities for afterschool, since this can offer you some new ways of enjoying a new start with some new people who share your interests.
- Make some fun plans for evenings, school vacations, and weekends, and this will mean you'll always have something that you can have on your radar that is positive. This will also keep your focus off the past.

- You are not the only one who has been bullied. If you see someone else who seems to be feeling isolated, try talking to them. You might be a part of the other person's healing process and you may heal in the process too.

Recovering from a bullying experience may take time and everyone will heal at their own pace. But if there have been months since it happened and you're not feeling better, you might want to speak with someone to help you.

What Exactly Is Cyber Bullying?

If you are being cyber bullied, you're certainly not alone. Cyber bullying in the UK is a growing trend and 7 in 10 (69%) of young people aged 13 and 22 have experienced cyber bullying with 20% of which had been very extreme. 37% of this experience bullying frequently. Child Line in the UK reports that 4,500 young people talked to them about online bullying last year. Another survey done by Slater and Gordon and the Anti-Bullying Alliance, found that over half of young people in England (55.2%) accept cyber-bullying as part of everyday life.

Cyber bullying happens when someone is using the Internet, text messages, social media, emails, online forums, instant messaging, and other types of digital technology to harass, threaten, or humiliate another person. Unlike the traditional types of bullying, cyber bullying doesn't need physical strength or contact face-to-face to happen. Cyber bullies come in every shape and size. Girls are more likely to be victims as well as bullies than boys. This is due to a number of reasons like low self-esteem, anger, frustration, and other suicidal issues. Often cyber bullying comes about because of other problems in the teenager's life like substance abuse, school performance issues, and delinquency. Almost anyone who has the Internet or a cell phone is able to cyber bully another person. They don't even have to reveal their identity. Cyber bullies are able to torment victims anytime during the day or night and they are able to follow the victims everywhere so the victim does not feel safe anywhere.

The Harmful Effects Of Cyber Bullying

The methods that teens use for cyber bullying can be as imaginative and varied as their technology. It will range from sending taunting or threatening messages by text, IM, or email to breaking into someone's account or stealing an online identity so that you are humiliated and hurt. Some of the cyber bullies can even create social media pages or websites to target you.

As happens with the traditional forms of bullying, both girls and boys do cyber bullying. The difference is that they have different ways of doing it. Boys will often do texting with messages that threaten to do you physical harm. Girls will spread rumours and lies, they will expose secrets, and exclude you from buddy lists, emails, or other kinds of electronic communication. Since cyber bullying is really easy to perpetrate, teenagers can often change their role, going from victim of cyber bullying to someone who is doing the cyber bullying.

How Could Cyber Bullying Affect Me?

Any kind of bullying often makes you feel helpless, angry, hurt, isolated, suicidal, and often leads to problems like anxiety, low self-esteem, and depression. In a lot of cases, cyber bullying sometimes ends up being more painful than the bullying that's done face to face for the following reasons:

- Cyber bullying is able to happen at any time, anywhere, even in the places where you usually feel safe like your own home. It often will happen when you don't expect it to happen, like during the weekend with your family around you. It often seems like there isn't an escape from the humiliation and taunting. Since they are unable to see how you are reacting, they'll often go a lot further in harassing or ridiculing you in comparison to face-to-face bullying.

- A lot of cyber bullying can be done anonymously, so you may not be sure who is targeting you. This may make you feel much more threatened, since they believe that online anonymity makes them less likely to be caught.
- Cyber bullying is able to be witnessed by lots and lots of people. Emails are able to be forwarded to countless amounts of people and social media posts are able to be viewed by just about anyone. When the bullying is very far-reaching, you are more humiliated.

How Can I Deal With Cyber Bullying?

If you have been targeted by a cyber-bully, you shouldn't respond to any posts or messages that have been written about you, even if they are really untrue or hurtful. When you respond, it's going to make your situation a lot worse. The cyber bully wants to provoke a reaction from you. Beat them at their game by ignoring them, which will make them lose their power over you.

It is also really important that you don't seek revenge on the cyber bully and become a cyber-bully yourself. It is only going to make the situation much worse and may mean legal consequences. If you would not say it face-to-face, do not say it on the Internet.

Do The Following Things To Respond To A Cyber Bully:

- **Save cyber bullying evidence.** Keep the abusive text messages or make a webpage screenshot. Then report the problems to an adult you trust, like a school counsellor, parent, or teacher. Never think you are a grass or a snitch. If you don't report the incidents, a cyber bully could become much more aggressive.
- **Report inappropriate messages of sex and harmful threats.** If you get messages that are highly inappropriate in a sexual way or someone's threatening you with bodily harm, tell the police. There may be legal consequences.

- **Be relentless**. Cyber bully rarely is limited to a couple of incidents. It's a lot more likely that you're going to be attacked as time goes by. So you have to keep on reporting the incidents. There's no reason that you should keep dealing with cyber bullying.
- **Prevent the cyber bully from communicating with you.** Block their email, block their cell number, and delete them from your social media contacts. Make sure you report the activities to their IP and to the websites they're using to target you.

Things To Remember If You're Being Cyber Bullied

- **You're not to blame.** This is NOT your fault. It doesn't matter what the cyber bully is saying or doing, you shouldn't be ashamed of what you're feeling or the person you are. The cyber bully has a problem, you don't.
- **Try to view the cyber bullying from another perspective.** The cyber bully is sad and frustrated and they want to control your feelings. Don't let them do that.
- **Do not dwell on it**. Don't make cyber bullying worse and dwell on it. Delete the cyber bullying messages and focus on your positive experiences. There are a lot of things that are great about you so you should be very proud of yourself.
- **Get some help**. Speak with a teacher, counsellor, or a parent. Speaking with a counsellor doesn't mean you have something to be ashamed of.
- **Learn to cope with your stress**. Finding some ways to relieve your stress, like doing your Morning Rituals (chapter 7), will make you much more resilient so you're not feeling overwhelmed by the cyber bullying. Muscle relaxation, breathing exercises, meditation, exercise, yoga and positive self-talk can help you to cope with the cyber bullying stress.
- **Spend some time doing the things you like**. When you spend time doing activities that are pleasurable for you –

such as sports, hobbies, spending time with your friends who aren't cyber bullies, the less time you will spend thinking about the cyber bully.

Get Some Support From Responsible People

Having people that you trust, that you are able to turn to in order to get support and encouragement is going to give your resiliency a boost when you are being cyber bullied. Reach out to those people who you trust like real friends and family and also find new friends. There are a lot of people who love you the way you are without changing yourself.

- Unplug the technology – Taking a break from your tablet, video games, iPod, cell phone, and computer will help you meet some new people.
- Find others who have similar tastes – Think about what you like doing and then find other people who like doing those things too. There are a lot of different ways that you can meet people, either through a club, hobby group, your church or through sports teams.
- Find a support group – There are a lot of support groups out there for people who have been bullied that you can join. If you are getting counselling through school, your counsellor may be able to suggest someone that you can talk to or a group that you can participate in.

For more help:

Get a FREE 80 Page Guide to Bullying & Cyber Bullying at
www.nobullying.com

UK: Call for more help 24/7 on 0808 800 5000 (adults) or call Child
Line on 0800 1111 (children) or email help@nspcc.org.uk
USA: Call LIFELINE at 1-800-273-TALK (8255) or visit
www.stopbullying.gov
Canada: Call Kids Help Phone 1 800 668 6868 or visit
www.kidshelpphone.ca
Australia: Call 1800 55 1800 or visit www.kidshelp.com.au

Chapter 6
Coping with Depression

When you are depressed, it may feel like no one knows what you are going through. But depression's really common in teens. You aren't alone and you're not hopeless, even though it may seem that way. Although it seems like your depression won't ever lift, it will eventually. With the right treatment and making healthier choices, the day can come much sooner.

Symptoms and Signs of Depression in Teens

It's really difficult to place into words the way depression often feels. Different people experience it in different ways. However, there are some common symptoms and problems that people who are depressed experience.

- You're constantly feeling sad, crying, angry, or irritable.
- Nothing feels fun and you don't even see why you should try.
- You have no self-esteem- you feel worthless, wrong, or guilty.
- You often feel you need more sleep or you don't get enough.
- You have unexplained, frequent headaches or other kinds of problems with your body.
- You're gaining or losing weight without even trying.
- You're unable to concentrate and your grades are falling.
- You feel hopeless and helpless.
- You're thinking about suicide or death.

Important note: If you are feeling this way, make sure that you talk to someone right away.

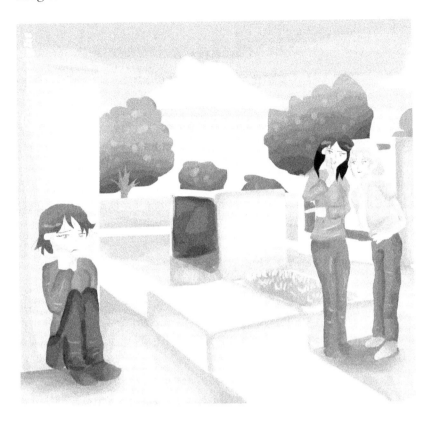

Why Is Teen Depression Increasing?

I find it very distressing that so many teenagers are affected by depression. Following is some information why young people are faced with this problem and some possible ideas how we can deal with it.

When I was a teenager twenty years ago depression in children was almost unknown. Now the fastest rate of increase in depression is among young people. This supports the research that most depression is not caused by gene imbalances.

What appears to be happening is changes in society where basic needs for friendship, fitness goals, and responsibility, are not being met. Teenagers are being fed a constant diet by the media of how they are supposed to look, sound and be, and told that this is important in life. Meaning is attached to what they have, or look like, rather than what they do, or achieve.

The popular reality TV programs and those who are supposed to be at the 'top' are hardly good examples of what we should be aiming for in life. As a teenager, you are under constant pressure to conform with your peers which can be often extremely strong. If you feel different, inadequate or deprived in some way, then depression may result, depending on how you deal with it.

Australian Teen Depression Study

In a recent study by the Queen Elizabeth Medical Centre in Western Australia, of 400 children aged 9 to 12, 16 were found to be clinically depressed, with 112 assessed as being vulnerable to future depression. Depressed children believed that happiness is achieved through the acquisition of fame, money and beauty. Happier teens tended to believe that feeling good comes from healthy attitudes to life and pursuing worthwhile life goals.

Many Studies Prove Good Personal Hygiene Improves Lives

Did you know that depression could be one of the effects of poor personal hygiene?
It's true. According to the Patient Education Institute, depression can stem from a general feeling of low self-confidence and self-worth brought on by poor hygiene and not feeling good about yourself.
A sudden change in your desire to take care for your personal hygiene and look smart and presentable could be a sign of serious mental illness.

This is another reason why I am so passionate about The Bum Gun bidet sprayer. There are so many more benefits to this amazing invention than just being better than toilet paper at cleaning your body.

Research has shown that when you neglect your personal hygiene you can find yourself ostracized from friends and family. Poor body cleanliness could affect you keeping your job, making friends or keeping your relationship going.

Poor hygiene can also limit you socially and make you feel alone, and prevent you from ever finding a partner if you are single.

Am I Depressed or Just In A Bad Mood?

Depression in teenagers can often be difficult to spot because of so many problems with growing up. In younger teens, depression may present as morbid preoccupation with death and dying. The child may exhibit extreme fear of being separated from a parent or parents and lose interest in participating in games with other children.

As you progress through your teen life, you will develop a stronger understanding that you are the most important one, and you don't have to try copy what your friends are doing.

I wanted to know how to help you through your teen life, with the beauty of hindsight. Worrying about all the wrong things can often lead to needless depression. Therefore, I carried out extensive research interviewing hundreds of young ladies and I found the following pointers kept coming up time and time again. I asked them "what do you wish you knew as a teenager which you think would have helped you through your teen life?"

These are the results below:
- Love yourself. If you don't, do whatever it takes to learn to love yourself. The only way you can grow up to be a strong woman and to have healthy relationships with anyone starts with loving yourself. To quote The Perks of Being a Wallflower, "We accept the love we think we deserve."
- In order to know what kind of man will be right for you in the future, you need to know who you are. Spend time with yourself. Be a kid. Have fun. Be single. Learn to enjoy your

own company before you spend a lot of your time with someone else.

- Most of the girls at my school seemed to look like Barbie dolls. They were pretty, tanned and had silky, blonde hair. I was a bit of a late starter and did not consider myself very attractive in high school. Plus, my skin was very pale. But I wanted to fit in to be considered pretty, too, so I started going on sunbeds and wearing fake tan all the time. But now I realise that fair skin is awesome and far healthier. Rock your own beauty.

- It's important to know whether you're putting energy into something that has the potential to pay off. This is one of life's biggest challenges. We often stay in dead-end situations way too long...hoping the situation will improve.

- While you're still young and have all this opportunity to learn, try not to limit yourself to what you, your parents or other people think you should focus on. Try different things. You might surprise yourself as to what you are good at or have passion for.

- Get out there. Do things. Meet new people. Create lots of memories and document them. Write a journal or take lots of photos. Even great memories fade over time.

- Surround yourself with lots and lots of books. Practice reading to build your stamina. There is not enough time in the world to learn, especially when you start late. I wish I had someone to tell me how important this was when I was a teenager.

- Coming from a very strict family and environment I felt we did not have access to enough sexual education. That was an issue that many would not talk about and it would have reduced a lot of unnecessary worrying to have been better informed about it.

- Keep in touch with your good friends. They are not easy to find.

When Your Depression Becomes Really Serious

It is evident that not only are teenagers becoming more depressed, they are also dealing with depression by killing themselves. The high rate of suicide may be due to the intense pressures felt by teenagers, coupled with a lack of life experiences that tell them that situations, however bad, will get better with time.

- Suicide amongst teenagers & young adults has increased 3 fold since 1970.
- 90% of suicide amongst teenagers had a diagnosable mental illness, depression being the most common.
- In 1996 suicide was the 4th biggest killer of 10 to 14 year olds, and the 3rd biggest killer of 15 to 24 year olds.

If your feelings are becoming so much that you're unable to see any kind of solution besides hurting yourself or other people, you must get some help now. But it can be hard to ask for some help when you are having strong emotions. There are suicide helplines that you can call and speak with someone completely anonymously.

Coping With Thoughts Of Suicide

There are a few things that you can do to help you with getting through this hard time.

- There is always something you can do, even if you're unable to see it – Many teens who've tried to kill themselves said they made the decision because they didn't believe there was another solution to their problems. At that time, they couldn't see any other way. Keep in mind that these emotions will pass, despite the way that you are feeling now. Time is a massive healer.

- Having these thoughts of hurting other people or yourself doesn't make you bad. Depression often makes you feel and think things that aren't normal for you. Nobody should condemn or judge you because of the feelings if you're brave enough to face them.
- If you can't control your feelings, tell yourself that you should wait 24 hours prior to acting on them – This is going to give you the time to truly think about things and distance yourself from those strong emotions. During this period, try speaking with someone motivating and understanding. Talk with one of your friends who is upbeat or call a suicide hotline. The hotlines are manned by people who understand what you are going through and they will not be judgmental. They will listen and be understanding. They are exceptionally well trained, super easy to talk to, and often had similar feelings when they were teenagers. That's why they want to help others, like you.
- If you're afraid you're out of control, don't be alone – Even if you're unable to speak about your feelings, remain in the public areas. Get together with your friends, spend time with family, go to the mall, go somewhere there are other people.

Above all else, don't do anything which could result in permanently damaging yourself or other people. Remember that your problem is temporary, but suicide is permanent. There is always help. You just have to find someone that you can talk to. You have to take that step.

Speak With A Trusted Adult About Your Depression

It may seem as if there isn't any way that your parents are going to be able to help, particularly if you feel they are always getting angry at you or nagging you. It may be that they are feeling frustrated since they do not understand what's happening or how they can help you.

A lot of parents do not know enough regarding depression in order to recognize it when their kids are hurting. You may have to tell them about how you are feeling and give them the information so that they know. Telling your parents that you are hurting will motivate them into helping you get the help you need.

Why You Should Accept And Share Your Feelings

It's often hard opening up about the way that you are feeling, particularly when you feel really depressed, ashamed, hopeless, and worthless.

It is very important to remember that everyone finds themselves with these kinds of feelings at some point in their lives. It is completely normal. It doesn't mean you are weak, flawed, or that you're not good. Accepting the feelings that you are having and talking about them with someone that you trust is going to help you with feeling less alone.

It doesn't matter what feeling you are having right now, remember that people care about you and love you. If you are able to find the courage to share your feelings about your depression, you are going to feel much better. Some people believe that talking about their sad feelings is going to make the feelings worse. But it is usually just the exact opposite. It's very helpful to talk to someone about your worries. They don't need the ability to fix the problems; they just have to be able to listen.

How You Can Feel Better – Tips For When You're Depressed

Depression is never your fault. You did not do anything to bring it on. You do have control over whether you feel better by choosing enjoyable things to do. Remain close with your family and friends, get out and take a walk, which will keep your stress levels down by avoiding stress triggers in your life. This can make a big positive impact on the way you feel.

It may be a good idea to get some therapy so that you are able cope while sorting out the feelings you are experiencing. Talk to your parents or a counsellor to see what options there are for treatment. If you are considering medication, do some research before you make a decision. Some of the antidepressants that are used by adults will often make teenagers feel worse. As always with medication, seek professional help first.

Don't Isolate Yourself

Spend some time with your friends, particularly those who are upbeat, active and who make you feel great about yourself. Don't spend time with those who are doing drugs or drinking alcohol, want you to do bad things, or who make you feel like you're insecure. It is also a great idea to reduce the amount of time you are surfing the Internet or playing online games.

Keep a Healthy Body

Making lifestyle choices that are happy can help your mood immensely. Things such as exercise and diet have been proven to help with lifting depression. Exercise actually releases a lot of endorphins and these make you happier instantly. You will actually receive an endorphin rush when you exercise. Physical activity will often work much better than therapy or medicine for your depression, so ride a bike, dance, or join a sport. Any kind of activity will help. Even regular brisk walks around the block, with your dog if you have one, can benefit you.

When it comes to food, a diet that is unhealthy and filled with processed foods can make you feel tired and sluggish, and this worsens your symptoms of depression. Your body needs minerals and vitamins. Be sure you're giving your brain what it needs by eating a lot of vegetables, whole grains, and fruits. Try to eat organic vegetables and fruits. Always remember to wash your fruit thoroughly. Speak with your school nurse, doctor, or parents about how you can be sure your diet is nutritious. If you have a gym membership or you're in a team at school, you can get great nutritional advice from the gym trainers or your coach at school.

Avoid Drugs And Alcohol

It may be tempting to use drugs or drink so that you are able to escape from the feelings you have and boost your mood, even if it's only for a little while. But substance abuse makes your depression worse. Using alcohol and drugs also can increase your suicidal feelings. Taking drugs and drinking alcohol is never a good idea, but especially when you're depressed.

If you have an addiction to drugs or alcohol, get help. You are going to need special treatment to help you with your problem, as well as the treatment for the depression.

Get Help If You're Under A Lot Of Stress

Worry and stress can really hurt you and they can lead to depression. Speak with someone at school if classes or exams feel overwhelming. If you have a problem with your health that you don't feel comfortable speaking with your parents about, like you think you're pregnant or you have a problem with drugs, go to a clinic or see your doctor. Health professionals are able to help you without approaching your parents and give you confidential guidance on treatment.

If you are dealing with friendship, family, or romantic problems, speak with one of the adults that you trust. There may be counsellors at school or you can ask your parents about seeing a therapist.

Helping Your Depressed Friend

Do you have a depressed friend? If one of your friends seems troubled or down, you may think that they are depressed. But is there a way that you can tell that it's not just a foul mood or a phase?

Here are some warning signs.

- She doesn't want to do your favourite things that you enjoyed doing in the past.
- She begins using drugs or alcohol or even hanging out with the wrong crowd.
- She stops going to her classes and her afterschool activities
- She says that she is ugly, worthless, bad, or stupid.
- She begins talking about suicide or death.

Teens who are depressed usually will rely on friends rather than parents or other adults to help them, so you may find yourself someone that they confide in. Even though this may seem like a big responsibility, there are things that you can do that will help.

- Encourage your friend to open up – Beginning a conversation regarding depression can really be daunting, but you might say something easy such as, "You really seem a bit down these days and not like yourself. I want to do something. How can I help?"
- Understand your friend does not expect you will have all the answers – The truth is your friend just wants a listener and someone to support them. When you listen and respond without being judgmental and are reassuring, you will help her.
- Encourage her to get some help – Urge your friend to speak with an adult. It may be really scary for her to admit that she has a problem to someone in authority. Offer to go with her if she would like, as moral support.

- Be with her through thick and thin – Depression may make her say and do things that are strange or hurtful. But she's going through a really hard time. Don't take anything personally. After she has received the help she needs, she's going to go back to being the person she used to be. While you're waiting, make sure that you have support that you need from your other friends and family. You need it like she does.

- If she's suicidal, speak up – If she's talking or joking about suicide, giving her possessions away, or she's saying good-bye, tell someone that you trust. Don't wait until something serious happens. You want to get some help for your friend and you need to do it really quickly. Even if she made you promise you wouldn't tell, she needs some help. It's a lot better to have her mad at you then to have a friend who is dead.

Helplines

If you're suffering and do not know where you should turn:
United States call the www.Nineline.org hotline for children and teens at 1-800-999-9999. It's free, confidential, and available from 4:00 PM to 8:00 PM, Eastern Time, seven days a week.
In the UK, call the www.Childline.org.uk helpline for children and teens at 0800 1111.
Australia, call www.Lifeline.org.aus 24-hour helpline at 13 11 14.
Canada, call www.KidsHelpPhone.ca helpline at 1-800-668-6868.

Chapter 7
Self-Development & Esteem Building

I wanted to share with you a story that happened to me in 1999. It was by far the most traumatic and devastating event in my life. My goal here is to help you understand that every difficult period of your life will pass, and your life will improve. Never give up during the difficult times in your life, and keep confident that Problems will blow over and your life will improve. I know it is a cliché but it's really true – time is a massive healer.

The Car Crash Which Changed My Life

... Mr Chang just blurted out without any warning "WHY DO YOU MAKE ME LOSE FACE?? Then I heard him thump the gas pedal hard as he tried to floor it!! The car was suddenly picking up speed, and I could see the speedometer needle increasing and increasing. We were suddenly doing 40 mph, then 50 mph, as I tried to plead with Mr Chang to slow down. But this guy was like a freak possessed. I have never ever experienced someone massively changing their mood so quickly, for no apparent reason. With the needle on the speedo still increasing ...My next action could be my last!!

My story began with me being manhandled from the overturned wreckage of a car at the side of a Bangkok highway. I remember being held by my wrists and ankles, similar to a lifeless corpse and being dumped into the back of a flat-bed pickup truck, a sorry excuse for an ambulance. But how did I get to this point?

At the time, I was working at a business college not far from my apartment. After a few months working at this college I was informed that we had a VIP guest arriving from the UK representing an English university they wanted to setup a joint program with. I was asked to look after him since we were both English. As it turned out, I didn't see much of him, as he had other colleges and universities to visit.

On the day of my accident, I was summoned to the Director's office and told it was our VIP visitor's last day. The owner of the school pleaded with me to join the company farewell dinner party that evening with the sole purpose of encouraging our visitor to choose our college. My boss also begged me to bring my girlfriend, as this would show our visitor that a happy family life was also achievable so far from home.

That evening we arrived at a swish 5 star hotel to find a group of old age, very rich looking purple haired Thai-Chinese ladies. We were given the standard swanky Chinese fare served on huge circular marble revolving tables. To be honest, I didn't like the food or the whole situation, as no one really spoke any English. Consequently, I could not wait to get the meal over with and get home.

Thankfully, the meal finally drew to a close, and it looked like everyone was getting themselves ready to head home. Suddenly, out of nowhere the husband of my boss, I'll call him Mr Chang, approached and insisted I join him and our visitor for a few drinks in an entertainment complex just down the road. His argument was that this 'grandma meal would not have given our guest much reason to choose our college.' I tried my best to get out of the invitation, but I was assured it would only be for an hour at the most. Reluctantly, I agreed to go for a short time, as we had work in the morning, nothing more than that.

So off we went; Mr Chang, our VIP visitor, another Thai teacher and my girlfriend. At the venue, admittedly, I did get the chance to do my part for the team and explain all the fantastic benefits of Thailand to our visitor, but we didn't see Mr Chang for most of the time. After about two hours he did appear though, paid the bill and told us it was time to go. We moved towards the lobby and waited for our driver, or whom I thought was our driver.

The next minute Mr Chang ushered us out of the door and it looked like he was thinking of driving. I asked him where his driver was, to which he replied that he was not needed as he had only had a couple of drinks. Still, this was definitely unacceptable to me, so I told Mr Chang that I would just catch a taxi, especially as I only lived a very short distance away. The response I got was not a friendly one. Mr Chang was very insistent that we all got in the car. I got the distinct feeling by the look on his face that if I persisted with my taxi idea then this would be very bad for my job. I had been in Thailand long enough to know that the Thai people can be very strange about what they might see as losing face. Reluctantly, thinking he'd be legally allowed to drive anyway, we jumped in the SUV and started the journey home.

Our distance back was only a few miles, but after a few minutes our visitor who was sitting on my right side in the back, said he was feeling sick. He told me he was not used to sitting in the back of a car, and asked me to ask the driver to slow down a bit. I told him to open the window a bit, and I leaned forward to explain the situation to Mr Chang. I noticed the speedometer had a reading of 35 mph. The next few moments would dramatically change all of our lives forever!!

Mr Chang just blurted out without any warning "WHY DO YOU MAKE ME LOSE FACE? I told you I had only 2 drinks!" Then I heard him thump the gas pedal hard as he tried to floor it! The car was suddenly picking up speed, and I could see the speedometer needle increasing and increasing. We were suddenly doing 40 mph, then 50 mph, as I tried to plead with Mr Chang to slow down. But this guy was like a freak possessed. I have never ever experienced someone to massively change mood so quickly, for no apparent reason.

The needle on the speedo was increasing and increasing to 60 mph, and then I saw the dial hit 70 mph. What was this guy on? And more importantly, what should we do to get out of this situation? I quickly told my girlfriend and our visitor to make sure they had their seat-belts on tight. Unfortunately, there was no seat-belt for the central position. In these kinds of life or death situations what can you do? Life seems to flash in front of your eyes at lightening pace! You kind of freeze, but your mind is also racing. Should I grab the driver in a headlock, and choke him out? Should I reach forward and pull hard on the hand-break? Both of these actions I thought might result in the SUV flipping over, or at least making the situation worse. The needle hit 75 mph and then 80 mph. I was screaming "Oh, my God" inside my head. This was just like a HBO movie but massively worse!! This was intensely real and happening right now!

What could we do? I looked up again and saw the speedometer needle hit 90 mph. Mr Chang suddenly started laughing and screamed out loud "look I can even do stunt driving!", and then began violently tugging the wheel from left to right. I knew right then we had seconds to go before an already nightmarish scenario was going to get even worse.

Suddenly, the car took off into the air, and then landed very hard with severe jolts!! With Mr Chang still yanking the steering wheel left and right it's a miracle the car didn't flip! Then I realized we had just driven over one of the Bangkok canals that run under many main roads. Mr Chang had managed to correct the vehicle this time, not that he was trying very hard to prevent a crash!! But, I knew there would be another canal coming very soon, and I just knew we wouldn't be so lucky the next time.

I knew I had to somehow wedge myself in to prevent being thrown from the car. I had very little to play with and only split seconds to act. I squashed up to my girlfriend behind the passenger seat thinking that would at least give me a barrier from being thrown forward, jammed my foot under the seat, looped my arm through my girl-friend's seat belt, and clenched her as hard as I could with both arms

– then BANG, we took off into the air again!!! But this time there was no recollection of a landing. Everything went black.

The next thing I remember was waking up as I was being carried by my wrists and ankles and being dumped into the back of a pickup truck. This was what I'd always called 'The Deadbody Snatchers,' Thailand's excuse for an ambulance service. These were volunteers in pickups who listen in to police radio with the intent of getting to the scenes of crashes first. They would then receive commissions from the hospitals where they take the crash victims.

My next recollection of anything was waking up in hospital. I tried to look around the room and work out where I was. I could make out what I thought was my girlfriend in the bed next to me, but facing away so I wasn't sure. I didn't have any power to call out to check. I was completely dazed and confused.

Then it HIT ME LIKE A FREIGHT TRAIN!! I had no feelings in my legs!! HELPPP I screamed out with what little strength I had. Two nurses appeared from somewhere. What's wrong with my legs?? What's wrong with my legs?? Where am I? The nurses explained I was in ICU, and that I should try to calm down. One ran off to fetch a doctor. The doctor told me that I'd had a car crash 3 days ago.

"WHAT ABOUT MY LEGS?? WHY CAN'T I FEEL MY LEGS??" I insisted. The doctor tried to assure me that it was normal to not be able to feel my legs after such a severe back accident. "A SEVERE BACK ACCIDENT?" What was he talking about? The doctor explained I'd had a very hard impact into my back, and that's why I couldn't feel my legs. But he said he thought the feeling would come back after a few days.

So I'm lying here thinking 'the doctor is telling me he thinks I'm not paralyzed but I've broken my back! Crikey! Do both mean I will never be able to walk again? It was then that I noticed that my pillow was covered in blood. I think this was too much shock for my system to handle and I just passed out.

The next few days were terrible, but mostly consisted of waking up for a few moments, being fed some medicine and falling back to sleep pretty quickly. I was just very drowsy and completely drained of all energy. But I did learn from a doctor that I had broken 4 bones in my back, and received two huge gashes to the back of my head, needing 22 stitches.

We Can Choose to be Powerful or Pitiful

Towards the end of the first week in hospital I woke and could still not feel my legs properly. It was then that I realised I might have to come to terms with the fact I would never walk again. I can't think of many devastating feelings worse than this, especially as I had always been so active in sports from a very young age.

Here I was waking up in an ICU in a foreign country with no one around me to help. There was no one to bring the obligatory grapes. The feelings and emotions were so intense that they are almost indescribable. I had left a loving family in the UK and a larger circle of friends than most people are lucky enough to have in life. Now I was lying in a hospital bed thousands of miles from home, lonely, feeling sorry for myself, thinking I was paralyzed. What was I thinking? Why did I leave my country? It wasn't supposed to be like this.

Eventually I realised that feeling sorry for myself was not going to make the situation any better. I'd seen filmstrips of brave young guys returning from war and going through all the rehabilitation steps to make the most of their lives. I wasn't dead, which was the main thing. And everything else after that would be a bonus.

I was brought up a Catholic, but I would not say I have ever been deeply religious. I have always tried to lead a good life though, and treat people the way I would like to be treated in return. Was this accident karma induced or just plain bad luck; wrong place, wrong time?

Then I began thinking that perhaps this accident was sent to test me, to build me up stronger, to face something even more challenging, something even greater than I'd ever faced before. It was then that I decided that this was where I would draw the line, I thought to my-self. We can always choose to be powerful or pitiful and I knew which one I wanted to choose. Therefore, I decided that this was the end of the sad, feel sorry for myself stage. It was time to fight on against all odds.

My Deal With God For The Chance To Walk Again

As I lay there, I was still deeply depressed and unsure if I was ever going to be able to walk properly again. What would life be like from now on without proper use of my legs, was still riding high in my mind. I felt like I needed a hand. Who else can help in this kind of situation? Well, if there is a God, then I need him right now, I thought.

So that's what I did. I made a deal with him. I wanted to say sorry for anything he thought I'd done wrong so far in my life, anything he thought I should have done better. I just wanted one gift from him. That I could walk again. I needed the strength and the willpower to get through all of my injuries.

But what was I going to give in return? I made a promise that if I could walk again, I would find a way to repay him. I needed to find something that could benefit as many people as possible. I truly wanted to make a profound difference in other people's lives. To do something so valuable, that generations would talk about what I had achieved for years to come, for decades, even for millenniums. Do something much greater than myself.

Crash, Battered, Broken, but not Defeated

After about 18 days I left the hospital rather suddenly. I still had a blood clot in my brain, hearing loss and a reduced bladder from infection. Doctors said I should not check out. But there were other concerns I needed to deal which I will explain at a later date. But finally getting home and lying down on my own bed again, after such a horrific ordeal, is indescribable, and here I was, finally back in my own apartment.

It was time for the next phase. Recovery and deciding what I was going to do to honour my side of the pact I'd made in the hospital. What was I going to do which was so valuable, that generations would benefit from for years after I had gone?

So there you have my story. I hope it wasn't too long, but this is the condensed version of all that actually happened. But I hope it will help you realize that life does prevent many difficult challenges for all of us to deal with. This whole experience was easily my most difficult challenge to come to terms with and ultimately beat. And I did succeed, and I came out a much stronger and a better person.
Keep reading for expert advice on how to deal with your self-esteem issues, and become a better person.

Self-Esteem Building

A lot of people have a problem with a low self-esteem and a lack of self-confidence. It is something that can happen at any age and to anyone, but it often happens to teenagers.
Low self-esteem is something that many teenagers have to deal with. If you have low self-esteem, you aren't alone. This chapter is going to:

- Help you learn what self-esteem is
- Help you deal with your feelings
- Provide you with useful actionable tips to build your self-esteem.

What Exactly Is Self-Esteem?

Nathaniel Branden, a doctor, who has expertise on the subject of self-esteem, has defined self-esteem as "the experience of being competent to cope with the basic challenges of life and of being worthy of happiness."

What this means is that when you have healthy self-esteem, you have as much esteem for yourself as you do for peers and friends. A lot of people have become so used to receiving negative feedback that we think more about our weaknesses instead of our strengths. A lot of times we are unable to enjoy the successes we have – it doesn't matter how big or small the success is – since we think that we are a failure.

Why Is Self-Esteem Important?

Having healthy self-esteem will play a role in just about everything you're doing. If you have high self-esteem, your relationships with adults and peers are better, you feel happier when you accomplish something, and you are able to better deal with failures and disappointment. You will be more likely to look for support and help from your friends and family. You're also much more likely to get good grades, set reasonable goals for yourself and accomplish them.

Another quote from Branden states, "Positive self-esteem is the immune system of the spirit, helping an individual face life problems and bounce back from adversity." From this you can see that having a high self-esteem will be vital during these difficult years while you're a teenager.

Everyone has a certain mental image of themselves and should understand the things we do well, and the weaknesses and strengths we have. This image is what plays a big role in developing a person's self-esteem. Healthy self-esteem is based on how you are able to accurately assess yourself and still be able to value and accept yourself unconditionally.

119

The daily experiences you have can affect the way that you feel about yourself. When you get a grade on a test, the ways that your friends treat you, things that happen in romantic relationships – can all impact your well-being temporarily.

If you have good self-esteem, the daily rollercoaster can fluctuate how you're feeling about yourself, but only to a small extent. But if you have low self-esteem, these kinds of fluctuations can make a huge difference and leave you feeling very dejected and full of negative self-awareness.
But there is good news – self-esteem is something you are able to work on so that it can improve.

Facts About Self Esteem

With so much information about self-esteem, it's important to know some of the facts about it. Here are some of the facts that you may not know about self-esteem that are important.

- Among students in high school 44% of the girls are trying to lose some weight.
- More than 70% of the girls between the ages of 15-17 stay away from normal activities every day, such as going to school, when they feel bad about the way they look.
- 75% of the girls who have low self-esteem said that they do negative activities, such as smoking, drinking, skipping classes, or engaging in eating disorders. This is high when compared with the 25% of the girls who have high self-esteem doing these activities.
- Teenage girls who have negative views of themselves quad-ruple their chances of having relationships with boys they regret down the road.
- The no.1 wish of all teenage girls is that their parents would improve their communication with them. This includes more open and frequent conversations.

- 7/10 girls believe they don't measure up or aren't good enough in different ways, including their school performance, looks, and their relationships with family members and their friends.
- The self-esteem of a girl is more related to the way that she views her body weight and shape rather than the amount she truly weighs.
- By the time they get to high school, just 29% of girls say they're happy with themselves. This means 71% of girls in high school aren't happy with the way they are.
- 1/3 of the girls from grades 9-12 believe they're overweight and 60% of them are trying to lose some weight.
- Just 56% of those in 7th grade like their looks.
- Teenagers who have low self-esteem are 1.6 times more likely to have problems with drugs than teens with normal self-esteem.

Expectations From Society

One of the biggest reasons that you might have low self-esteem is because of the unfair expectations that society places on you. There are three different ways that society places expectations on you.

Peer Expectations

Most people have been involved in relationships with people who are influential. These kinds of people are in your social circle, in your class or they are acquaintances. They are close enough so that they're able to manipulate the thoughts and feelings you have so that you think the way they think.

When you are influenced by your friends it can go one of two ways. It can go the correct way many times. An example of this would be when you see your friends excelling and you feel motivated so that you can do well too. You hadn't been quite as good as they were and you were motivated to improve yourself and work harder.

However, there are some times when you feel like you are an outcast. This kind of anxiety is something you may feel on a lot of levels – whether it's material possessions, appearance, or in your social circle. Wanting to be noticed because you are popular or beautiful is something that is very difficult for many people these days, and often leads to lowering your self-esteem.

Parental Expectations

It's common knowledge that parents compare us with other children. But think about the story of Cinderella. The shoe which fits one specific person will not fit another person. Unfortunately, it's rare that we apply this principle to real life.

In addition to these expectations that come from your parents, we make matters a lot worse when we give into or agree to these conformity desires. When you mould yourself to someone else's dreams or expectations for your life, this can cause you to be unhappy and can cause very big problems with your self-esteem.

Society

The pressures that society puts on all of us have been around for many years. For hundreds of years, people have sought to be better than other people and it's something that we have had to deal with for a long time.

Times are now changing, and people are turning out to be a lot more inclined and independent on hearing their individual voice. In spite of this, there are still a lot of people who find themselves caught up in the transition. So they don't know the way to deal with the opinions, critiques, and views of society.

This is a big reason why a lot of teenagers just like you might have low self-esteem. Unrealistic and over-exaggerated views of what perfection means is what creates problems for many people mentally, emotionally, and sometimes physically. Many teenagers run around and try adhering to every perfection definition that exists and that has existed. After they've failed at trying to be perfect, they think they're failures.

Traumatic Pasts

This can be something that ranges from the first time you failed a test at school to an experience when you might have been molested. These types of unacknowledged trauma sources will often pile up, causing irrefutable damage.

If you were bullied when you were in grade school because you were overweight, this trauma might still be continuing. Even if you have lost weight, you may still think that you are still fat and you are looking for ways to make yourself look a lot thinner.

This feeling that you're a failure, when actually you're hurting yourself, can be because of a low self-esteem. The first time you allow someone to make fun of you causes you not to have any faith in what you can do. When you don't have faith in yourself, this can cause you to have neurotic behaviour.

Self-Consciousness

Remember the time you didn't compete in a sporting event because you were sure you'd lose? Chances are that you have dreamt over and over again that you had competed and that you lost and that everyone was laughing at you. You start believing that everybody's watching you and waiting for you to mess up. You also think they're watching all the moves you make, all the mistakes you make, and that all of your mistakes are following you. You think that every time you make a mistake it's going to follow you and leave a scar which will stay forever.

You are afraid that you're different, that everyone's staring at you, or that people are going to treat you like you're from another planet. These are the things that keep you from experiencing new things. This fights with the need to be liked and popular. This kind of contradiction can make you slowly insane as you're driving right into a crowd.

Body Image

This can have a huge impact on your personal self-esteem since the idea that in order to be accepted, loved, and happy you have to be beautiful is constantly being sent by the media and society.

It's really important to create a positive view about your looks when you're a teenager because your mind is still developing at this point. This makes it easier to establish positive patterns of thinking. If you wait until you are older, it will be harder for you to break your negative thinking, although it's not impossible.

The ironic thing is that your teenage years are some of your life's most influential years but they are also probably the time in your life that's the most superficial. A lot of your world socially is going to be effected by the level of attractiveness you think you have.

It will take a great deal of maturity for you to be able to rise above these superficial expectations so that you're able to accept yourself the way you are. Confidence will really come from inside of you and you will need to consciously work at it if you want to become more confident. In addition, the way you look is constantly changing as you become a woman, so the way that you look now will not be the finished product of the way you'll look when you have finished growing. But you need to learn to accept yourself and you will have a much happier life. The good news is that this chapter is loaded with fantastic advice, so keep reading.

Family Life

A big reason that a lot of teenage girls have low self-esteem is the family and home life they have. How you view life can also make a difference in the way you view yourself. If you are in a family that has a healthy outlook on your body image and provides you with unconditional love and positive feedback, you will likely have healthy self-esteem. On the flip side, if you have been abused at all by someone at home or you are or were always put down, it can be harder to have a good outlook of yourself.

In your home, your self-esteem's biggest influence is your parents. When your mother's constantly worrying about her weight or the way she looks or her self-esteem is low, that can affect the way you look at yourself. You will learn these things from her and the chances are that you are going to have the same concerns about yourself. She'll also be concentrating on her issues rather than helping you create some healthy self-esteem for yourself.

Your mother isn't the only one who is going to affect your self-esteem. There are studies which show that the emotional state and self-esteem of a girl will be influenced greatly by her dad. Receiving some reassurance from your dad that you're important as you're growing and changing is going to give your self-confidence a huge boost.

Sometimes a girl doesn't have a father living in their home or they have a dad who ignores them or talks to them like they're not important or worthy. These kinds of girls often aren't able to love themselves and don't have good self-esteem. If you're in this kind of situation, keep in mind you're not to blame. When you are able to overcome your low self-esteem you will end up much stronger because of it.

Authority Figures That Were Disapproving

If you've encountered a lot of people in your life such as teachers or coaches who said that the things you were doing weren't good enough, how are you going to have a self-image that's positive? If you were criticized excessively no matter what you did or how hard you were trying, it is really hard to feel comfortable and confident as you grow. The shame that was forced on you because you perpetually failed can be very painful.

Conflicting Authority Figures

When caregivers such as parents fight or make one another feel bad, children absorb those distrustful situations and negative emotions that were modelled. It's disorganizing, overwhelming, and scary. This type of experience also can happen when one of the parents is acting uncharacteristically or they are deeply distraught because of the loss of a close friend, a major problem at work or fighting financial problems. If you have been subjected to a lot of conflicts between your parents, it may feel like you've contributed to those fights or the painful circumstances of a parent. This can cause you to have low self-esteem.

Bullying When Parents Are Unsupportive

If you have had trouble with bullying and your parents aren't supportive and don't listen to you, this can lower your self-esteem. If you are already feeling unsafe in your home and you are being bullied at school, you are going to have low self-esteem. You may feel hopeless, abandoned, and feel like you don't have any worth. You may also feel as if anybody is being friendly to you it is only out of pity, since you think you're worthless. You also might feel as if anybody in your life can't be trusted. Without a supportive life at home, effects of bullying are often magnified and can erode the quality of your life miserably.

Bullying With Over-Supportive Parents

If you have parents who are indiscriminately and overly supportive, it also can make you feel as if you're unprepared for the world. Without a reason to develop a thick skin, it often feels challenging and sometimes shameful if you view yourself as not being able to face life's challenges outside your home. When you have this perspective, it may be that you feel unprepared and you're deeply ashamed to admit this ugly, dirty spirit to anyone, even your parents. The reason for this is because you feel the need like they should be protected from pain that they'd feel if they discovered the truth.

Rather, you try to hide this painful secret about what's happening to you. This shame may be overwhelming and can cloud your judgment. Eventually it may seem as if the opinion that your parents have conflicts with the opinion the world has of you. It may make you want to cling to the things that you know and question how valid your parents' view is. You may then feel as if you're worthless and that you're a victim and you deserve ridicule.

Bullying With Parents Who Aren't Involved

If your caregivers are occupied when you were being bullied, downplay what happens to you, or don't stand up for you when you needed their help, you may feel like you don't deserve being noticed, that you don't deserve attention, and angry that you were short-changed. When you feel like the world's not safe, pain and shame can be brutal. These kinds of feelings might also happen if your parents are going through a lot of problems, since the things that you are going through aren't being noticed. If your home feels chaotic, it may be really hard to tell your parents about your problems. You might isolate yourself and retreat to your room.

Academic Challenges, No Caregiver Support

One of the biggest reasons that a lot of teenagers have low self-esteem is academic problems at school. If you are having problems in school and you are getting further behind and no one notices, you may feel like you're stupid. If you are having trouble in school and your parents aren't offering you the help that you need, you are going to feel that you are dumb and that there's nowhere you can turn. You may be embarrassed to ask someone to help you because you feel as if you are not worth the time.

Belief Systems

Sometimes a religion may make you feel as if you are always sinning. If you are in a family that follows this type of religion, this could be similar to feeling as if you're living with a person in authority who is always disproving of you. Whether this type of judgment is coming from a belief system or an authority figure, it can often evoke conflict, guilt, self-loathing, and shame. Many belief systems will offer you two paths – one of them that is completely good and one of them that is all bad. If you are between these two paths, you could be feeling wrong, confused, shameful, fake, disappointed, and disoriented a lot of the time.

In What Ways Can I Improve My Self-Esteem?

Long before you can start improving your self-esteem, you have to believe that it is possible to change. This change may not happen easily or quickly, but it's something that will happen if you consciously allow it to.

14 Tips To Improve Your Self Esteem

Here are some tips that you can use to improve your self-esteem:

1. **Dream big with unshakable confidence** – Become an unshakable optimist. Talk about and think about only the things you want. Your potential is unlimited. You CAN do it, so tell yourself you can. Optimism is the one quality most associated with success and happiness than any other.

2. **Stop thinking about yourself in a bad way** – Instead, celebrate the achievements and strengths you have. Write down 5 things you are able to do well and put it on the mirror in your bedroom. Repeatedly read this list until you're able to say the things without even thinking about them. Remember the list when you're feeling low. It will help you feel much better. Also, incorporate this list in your Morning Rituals.

3. **Be wary of perfectionism** – Rather than trying to be perfect, aim to accomplish things. The desire to be perfect will trap and burden you with needless stress.

4. **Overlook mistakes** – Rather than seeing mistakes as mistakes, see them as opportunities for learning. Everyone makes mistakes. See the mistakes as only feedback, and then use that feedback to keep improving the next time.

5. **Don't put yourself down** - Stop beating yourself up because of your weaknesses. Everyone has some weaknesses, and no one can do everything well. Better to focus on doing a few things really well, than doing many things averagely.

6. **Try out new things** – When you try new things, be proud of the things you have learned how to do.

7. **Begin doing things for others** – Do volunteer work, mentoring other students, or even tutoring. When you believe you're able to help people, you will have much better self-esteem.

8. **Understand what you're able to change. Then accept the things that you can't change**. You can't change things like body type, race, and height. But things like smiling more and your weight are things that you can change. If you want to lose weight, look on the internet like YouTube for an exercise plan and a healthier diet. Try to smile more by practicing while looking in your mirror and give yourself the challenge to smile at least 25 times per day.

9. **Stop negative self-talk** – Most people's worst enemy is themselves. Negative self-talk is when you are hearing negative thoughts going through your brain. One of the ways that you can stop these thoughts is to place a rubber band on your wrist. Every time you have a negative thought, snap the rubber band. After you have done this for a while you will reprogram your mind to avoid negative thoughts.

10. **Have a 2 minute self-appreciation timeout**. This is a very simple and important habit. If you spend just two minutes on it every day for a month then it can make a huge difference. Take a deep breath, slow down and ask yourself this question: What are 3 things I appreciate about myself?

11. **Exercise daily** – When you exercise, you boost your endorphins, and these are the natural opiates in your body which make you feel good. When you exercise every day, you will ease your stress, you will feel much better, and the more effective you will become. Keep in mind no one has

the power to make you feel bad – No one has the power to do that, only you.

12. **Think about the time you tried something new the very first time**. You will often feel nervous when you try something new and you will feel that you can't do it. When you feel less than confident again, remembering that these feelings are normal will help get you through.

13. **Do something you've put off** – This can be something as simple as calling or writing to a friend, tidying up your bedroom or your garage for your parents, or even washing the windows. When you make a decision and follow through, you are in charge.

14. **Talk to someone** - In the cases in which self-criticizing habits and emotional pain are long lasting or deep, you might want to speak to a therapist or a school counsellor for help. You can also talk to your doctor. Professionals in mental health are able to help you change negative behaviours and teach you positive ones that can help with boosting your self-image.

Read this chapter again every time you have self-doubt.

Do Something You're Good At

There are things that you are good at. There are a lot of things that you can do. You can swim, run, dance, cook, write, paint, or anything else. Make sure that you're doing something that holds your attention. When you have to focus on something positive it is easier to forget about everything else. You are going to feel accomplished, capable, and competent, which are all wonderful antidotes to the problem of low self-esteem.

Give Yourself Time To Relax

When you are feeling anxious, and low in confidence, one thing that you should do is to quit thinking and properly relax. Sometimes this can be done by exercising, other times it can be done by becoming involved in a mind-occupying activity. But having the ability to relax anytime you want to will be a great life skill. It's also a great idea to try self-hypnosis, meditation, or even Tai Chi. When you are relaxed properly, your brain will be less emotional and the memories of good events can work to your advantage.

Think About All Your Achievements

This may be hard in the beginning, but as time goes by you're going to have a list of memories that boost your self-esteem. These don't have to be monumental, like writing a huge novel.

These are things such as:

- Learning to ride a bicycle despite being really nervous at first
- Helping your team win something
- Doing well on a test even though you thought that you didn't do well.

Things Not to Say to Someone With Low Self Esteem

If you have a friend who has low self-esteem, there are things that you should never say to them. Here are some of the things that you shouldn't say if you know anyone who has low self-esteem.

After They Have Broken Up With Their Boy-friend/Girlfriend

"You are so wonderful, you are going to find another person soon."

When your friend isn't feeling very optimistic following a breakup, expressing optimism might not be the best idea. If your friend is upset because they're apart from their loved one, saying this won't help. It often will feel false and dismissive.

"It's not a big deal, you will move on soon"

This is another phrase that may seem dismissive. It minimizes the pain that the person is feeling, even if you're only trying to make someone feel better.

"You had a wonderful learning experience."
It's true that finding a silver lining in this type of experience could seem to be helpful. However, even if this is true, it's not something that you should point out.

When the person feels lonely

"Why don't you try doing _____ to meet other people?"
This really is well-intentioned. When you say this, you're encouraging the person to become proactive by giving them a few solutions to their problem of loneliness. But sometimes the person isn't looking for a solution. They can find the solutions themselves. They know how they can meet people. Your friend might just want you to understand how they feel.

After they received a bad test grade
"It is just one test, so it does not matter."
Simply because you are saying something doesn't matter, it doesn't mean that it doesn't make a difference to your friend.

Things You Can Do to Help Someone With Low Self Esteem
Now that you know the things that you should never say to someone who has low self-esteem, let's look at the things that you can do to help a friend who has low self-esteem:

- **Get them involved.** Try getting your friend involved with other people. This is going to help them see they're able to make positive contributions to people, events, and causes.
- **Provide them with positive feedback.** Tell them about their assets, strengths, and accomplishments. This is going to show them you think they're important since you remember the things they've done. It's also going to help them learn how they can reinforce their behaviour positively.
- **Express your concern and care.** Tell your friend how you care about them and that you appreciate that they're a part of

your life. This is going to show them that they belong in your life because you want them to be around.

- **Encourage them.** Try getting your friend to learn something new. Applaud their attempts, successes, and even their failed attempts.

- **Laugh with your friend rather than at them**. Give your friend some help so that they're able to laugh on their own and your own mistakes by locating the humour (when it's appropriate) they have in life.

- **Listen when they talk.** Let your friend express their feelings by providing them with your undivided attention when they're talking to you. This is going to show their opinions are important to you and their concerns should be heard, understood, and that you want to pay attention to what they are saying. Don't ignore them and answer text messages or play a game on your phone. Stay focused and show you care.

- **Give them compliments**. When they say or do something considerate, sweet, funny, sincere, or anything else, take it in a gracious manner and give them an appropriate response.

- **Don't get angry quickly.** It's going to be easy to become annoyed with people who are always self-depreciating, but they're in a really fragile position at the moment. Getting angry at them is going to make things a lot worse. If you become angry, they'll feel like you're against them and it will make it worse.

- **Think about their feelings**. When you see someone is sad, sometimes you will stay away from them or pretend the person doesn't exist. But this is not what you should do. If your friend has low self-esteem they need to know that you care about them because they likely feel as if no one else does. For example if you see your friend crying. You go over and ask them what is wrong. They tell you to go away. Don't go away. If you do that, it's going to make your friend feel much worse. Sit with them and give them comfort, even if they're not saying what is bothering them.

- **Discover what they're struggling with.** There's something that's giving them trouble. It might be their confidence, social fear, feeling lonely, problems with bullying, or feeling like they don't fit in. Try find out the reason they're feeling like they are, what they're feeling, and exactly what they want.
- **Understand they may be bitter.** When people take emotional beatings, they might be bitter. You should be gentle and compassionate since most people who put themselves down and they will generally be defensive.
- **Take care of what you're saying.** People who have low self-esteem are extremely vulnerable and sensitive in those areas that make them insecure. You might shrug off a snide remark, but someone that has low self-esteem might take it to heart and crumble. Just like you would not expect a toddler to shake off an injury or bruise, it's the same thing with someone who has low self-esteem with taunting jokes or nasty comments.

Self-Esteem Conclusion

Having a healthy self-esteem is important for you, since it can affect the way that you act and how you see yourself. Low self-esteem can lead to many problems that you may not know about. If you are having trouble with self-esteem, remember this chapter and the things that I have discussed with you. I don't have all the answers but hopefully I've given you some helpful advice which you can use to improve the quality of your life. Remember, if you have low self-esteem you aren't alone. Also remember that there are things that you can do to help yourself feel better and to give you a much better outlook on life.

My 8-Step Morning Ritual

"YOUR LIFE IS AN EXAMPLE OF YOUR DOMINANT THOUGHTS!!"

One of the greatest boosts I have had in my life was when I discovered the power of Morning Rituals. You might have heard that how you start your day, is how you end your day. I feel it is essential to start every day as you mean to go on. If you decide to join me and to begin doing this morning ritual I promise you that you will feel a massively better and it will give you an awesome start to every day. The whole idea about having a morning ritual is to empower you to have every opportunity to be at your best, and you will get much more from every day and from your entire life.

Here are my steps to start your day in a very positive and empowering way. Please feel free to modify my morning ritual to suit yourself. But perhaps start out for your first month how I have laid out here so you can have a proper understanding of a workable Morning Ritual.

Step 1: Drink Water

After oxygen, the next most important thing that our bodies require is water. It is a little known secret that having the first glass of water as soon as you wake up has many therapeutic benefits. This traditional Ayurvedic treatment has benefits for conditions that range from asthma, pain to even cancer.

- 70% of your body is water
- Your brain cells contain about 85% of water.
- 75% of your muscles is water
- Your bones contain about 25% water
- 82% of your blood consists of water.

Once you wake up, you are massively dehydrated. Your body is crying out for nourishment from water. That's why the first part of my morning ritual is always to drink a big cup of water as soon as I wake up. I try to drink at least 1 big cup of water, 2 if possible to ensure that I'm fully hydrated.

Step 2. Priming & Meditation

The next part of my ritual is something I do called Priming, and meditation.

Priming is something that I learned from Master Coach Michael Bolduc, which is a 10-minute exercise that primes you for gratitude and strength. It's something that I try to do every morning while sitting on my bed.

Here's how it works

1. Sit upright on your bed with your legs crossed and your eyes closed.
2. Take 30 really deep, strong breaths in and out through your nose, while raising your hands up and down. Make sure to inhale and exhale through your stomach and do it rapidly.
3. Think of 3 things in your life that you are grateful for. Think of anything, however big or small. It could be something like being grateful for the weather, or the comfort of your bed. Find gratitude in all of the things in your life.
4. Do another 30 explosive breaths in and out through your nose.
5. Think of 3 things you want to achieve in your day ahead. It can be small things like getting to school on time, or doing well in a test. It can be anything you want. Focus and visualize those 3 things. See them as if they are real.
6. Do another 30 explosive breaths in and out through your nose.
7. Next, spend a few minutes meditating as you feel really peaceful sitting in this position.
8. Last, finish by thanking your creator, while asking for any healing or power for that day. Open your eyes.

This process has been fantastic in helping me start the day in a totally uplifting way.

Breathing is an important step in any morning ritual, as oxygen is the most important thing that the body requires from a health perspective. By doing this exercise, I am also consciously focusing on my breathing and taking in deep breaths. This helps to cleanse and vitalize the cells of my body.

Step 3. Incantations

During my 7-minute workout (see no.4 below) I focus on conditioning my mind through incantations. This is another strategy that I learned from the Master Coach Michael Bolduc. Incantations are positive statements said out loud with emotional intensity. When you speak things out loud with emotion, you begin to condition your nervous system into believing what you're saying. There's a lot of power in this in shaping your own beliefs and emotions.

Examples of Possible Incantations

Here are some examples of incantations, but you will need to create your own.

"I, Greg Noland, see, hear, feel & know that I am a confident person, and my purpose in life is to be active, contribute and make a difference in people's lives!"

"I, Greg Noland, see, know, hear, and feel that I am healthy and energetic!"

"I am a determined person who is achieving all my goals to live my ideal and extraordinary life"

My Life Goals

I also like to combine my life goals with my incantations to get really pumped. I believe that focusing on your goals every day is an extremely important part of achieving them. This makes sure you are always reminded of them and focused on what you want in your life.

For example, here are some examples of goals you could set for yourself:

"I will get my highest score on this upcoming test!"

"I will complete my new exercise routine every day as soon as I wake up!"

"I will make my parents proud, today, tomorrow and every day!"

Step 4. 7 Minutes of Exercise

The next most important part of my morning routine is to get moving. It's short enough that it won't impact the rest of your morning routine and long enough to shake off any sleepy feelings. Remember too, that movement is one of the easiest and fastest ways to change your state.

Currently, I am using this routine shown on this website, www.7-min.com but you can use any exercise routine you find, or design your own 7 minute burst of energy.

Moving your body can mean going for a walk, running, dancing, jumping up and down, or anything that gets your blood flow moving.

Step 5. Empowering Questions

During the next part of my morning routine, I will direct my focus by asking myself empowering questions. I often like to do this part while I am brushing my teeth and while I'm taking my shower.

Whatever you focus on you feel. By directing your focus, you will change your state. The most powerful way of doing this is through questions.

Here are some of the questions that I ask myself every morning:

What am I most grateful for in my life right now?

What am I happiest about in my life right now?

What am I excited about in my life right now?

What am I passionate about in my life right now?

What am I committed to achieving today?

Who specifically can I help today?

How specifically am I going to help someone today?

Step 6. Breakfast: Start your day out green.

You'll be shocked at the amount of unstoppable levels of energy you can get from a green smoothie. I've found that blending one apple, one banana, one orange, a handful of spinach, half of a cucumber, any juice or coconut water you have, a few of ice cubes and some flax seed for about a minute is cheap, easy, extremely energizing and mega healthy. Try it.

Step 7. Plan Your Day

I usually plan my day before I go to bed. I have a pad beside my bed and review the goals I have for that day, week and month. During breakfast I like to go over my plan so it is fresh in my mind for the whole day. I often write out 3 goals for the day on a separate piece of paper and put that in my pocket. Then throughout the day I will take this out and read over my goals again. This helps me to stay focused on my main goals, and helps me take action on my goals to have the biggest impact in my life.

When you talk about something, it's a dream. When you envision it, it's exciting. When you plan it, it's possible. But, when you schedule it, it's real - Tony Robbins

Step 8. Empowering Beliefs

I have a list of empowering beliefs that I like to choose from to read out loud. The key is to consciously choose what you WANT to believe and begin to condition it daily by saying it out loud. If it is not possible to say these empowering beliefs out loud, for example if you are on the school bus, you can still go over them in your mind.

For example, some of the empowering beliefs I use to condition myself at the start of everyday are:

"I love my life!"

"What I do today, shapes my day and creates my tomorrow."
"Nothing is better than eating and being healthy!"
"I am generous and loving to all my friends and family!"

Now Get To It – Design & Build Your Morning Ritual

These are the 8-steps that I follow everyday as part of my morning ritual that allows me to be unstoppable every day. Of course, you can modify your morning ritual to keep it fresh and exciting.
I ask you to commit to trying your morning ritual for the next month. Try it every morning without fail. If you forget, or wake up late, still try to do some of it. But really try your best to complete your full ritual every morning for the next month. Go to bed 15 minutes earlier, and set your alarm to wake you up 15 minutes earlier than normal.

In the beginning write out step-by-step process and put it somewhere that you can view it every day. I promise you that you will feel awesome and much more confident, even a complete new person if you commit to it for the next month. You will be more productive than ever before and achieve much more. You will be healthier and more energetic than you ever thought possible. Your relationships with your friends and family will improve. Most importantly of all, you will be happier and more fulfilled.

I would be very grateful if you could email me and tell me how your Morning Ritual has positively impacted your life – please email me at greg@omgteenbookseries.com and let me know about your ritual.

"A Dream Life Is A Vision Which You Desire Most With Enough Compelling Reasons TO DO WHATEVER IT TAKES"

Chapter 8
Successful People Are Responsible

Responsibility can cover many things, such as being sensitive to other people's feelings, anger management and selflessness as opposed to selfishness. When you were a kid, you were the center of the universe. But now you are a teenager and become more responsible, you must be accountable and responsible for your own actions, be they good or bad. I feel responsibility is important because it means that, not only do you feel you are more mature and dependable, but other people see it as well. By being responsible, not only do you show other people that you can be dependable, but you show yourself too.

In this chapter I will cover some different areas of responsibility that will help you become a better person when you understand this quality more, and make steps to improve yourself.

Being Responsible at School

Responsibility is essential in all the parts of your life, but perhaps one of the most important parts is being responsible at school. Your days at school help you with learning and creating the habits that will help you enjoy the rest of your life.

This chapter will cover:
- Organization Tips
- Note Taking Tips
- Homework Tips
- Tips for Writing a Paper
- Study Tips
- Tips for Taking Tests

Being focused and learning the skills to get things done doesn't just mean getting good grades. It can help you with being successful throughout your life. Becoming organized and completing your work is going to help you in all aspects of your whole life.

Becoming Organized

The level of your success in high school starts with being as organised as possible. It is very difficult to study, meet deadlines and do well in your exams if all your notes and subjects are all jumbled together.

I great habit I discovered in high school was using a business box file to keep class information and assignments together in one place. I organized each folder based on subject, and colour coded them. Every time I had a loose document, course hand-out, graded assignment, paper or fact sheet, I would file it away in the right folder, so I never lost important information, and I knew exactly where to find it when I needed it later. I think this one technique saved me many wasted hours of searching at high school. In fact I still use this awesome technique in my business life to this day.

There is no need to stuff loose papers into your school bag or carry different spiral notebooks for each of your classes. One simple way is to follow the idea of the box folder at home and take a colour coded ring binder with different sections to school. When you get home after school, you can transfer these notes to your master box folder.

Also, a really good habit to get into is writing out all your notes when you get home. This gives you the opportunity to check whether you understand everything, do further research for better understanding and add in more details. This is going to take more time, but it's a great skill for studying since it gives you a far deeper understanding of the subjects.

There is no perfect solution for being organised, but if you are like most people you won't already have your own system for being organised so try my system. If that doesn't work for you, try another system. Whichever you decide on, the system needs to work well. If the system doesn't work, change your system around until you've found what will work.

Always Organise Yourself in Advance

If I can give you one single piece of advice, which will give you the best chance of succeeding at high school, and indeed well into your adult life, then it has to be the power of mastering procrastination. So many people bring so much stress on themselves by thinking "they'll do it later". But what usually happens is they forget about the assignment or task, and then they are forced to rush through a piece of poor work at the last minute.

I was just like this too. I often thought I had a handle on the situation and I usually had an imaginary time slot in my mind when I'd deal with each assignment. But you know what, that time slot always came and past. Does that happen to you?

I would always have the best intensions to complete the work on time, but something else always came up. As a result I often had to do an all-nighter to get the work done. Then the next day I would be so tired at school that I'd get further behind.

It wasn't until after my high school days that I discovered the skills of successful time management. When I read 'The 7 Habits of Highly Effective People' by Steven Covey my life changed. Suddenly I had the knowledge and skills to live a much more productive and stress free life. I also urge you to read 'Getting Things Done – The Art of Stress Free Productivity' by David Allen.

For now though, try these 3 Time Management Tips

1. Do the most important thing first
2. Concentrate on ONE particular task at a time, and FINISH it, before moving on
3. Block off your time in 50 minute chunks and stick to your plan

More than likely, it will be just you regarding working on your school assignments. It may feel great when you are in charge, particularly if you're good at it. Never leave your assignments until the day before. If you do, you are going to have to work a lot harder and you won't get good scores either. Stress will make it difficult to remain focused so that you're doing well.

Make deadlines, and stick to them. When each semester starts, create a calendar and put due dates on it. Make sure that you know when your main assignments are due and if your teacher doesn't tell you, ask about them. Also write the format the assignments are going to be in, such as presentation, group work or report. Setting some clear goals for yourself will help you remain focused.

When you are organizing the calendar, remember these questions:

- What is going to be the end project?
- When do the parts of the assignment have to be finished? The deadline.

When you answer quality questions, it will let you organise your assignments by difficulty level, completion time, and due dates.

Put non-academic commitments onto your calendar, like drama rehearsals, team practices, and others. This is going to help you with seeing when other things might create a crunch time during your semester. You should block out specific time during the evenings to complete your assignments. In addition, while you are working, you should stay focused and work. That means, turn off your phone, and if you are working on your computer, only have the necessary programs open. Limit all distractions. Chatting with friends should be done only in your 15 minute break times.

Challenge yourself with miniature deadlines for project stages – things like planning, researching, first draft, next draft, review, edit, and final draft creation.

Keep To A Tight Schedule

Figure out how to enforce the deadlines that you set for yourself. For instance, are you going to reward yourself when you meet them? Ask your parents or friends to check on how you are doing on your mini-deadlines. This way you are less likely to put things off. If you ask your parents, remember they are not nagging you. They are just doing what you asked them to do. Your friend can also act as an accountability coach to remind you of the goals you have set for yourself.

If you have a hard time with meeting your deadlines but you're attempting to improve your organization and study skills, speak with your teacher. Your teacher can help you with creating reasonable goals for a certain test or project.

Forgot About An Assignment?

If you find you have forgotten about an assignment, and you have a limited turnaround time, try to keep from freaking out. Use breathing exercises for becoming focused and calm. Then create an approach for tackling your work. Making a daily or hourly deadline calendar is a good idea if it helps with time structure.

Note Taking Tips

Write down the important facts – If your teacher writes notes on the board, this is a bonus, as it's easy for you to copy those notes down. If they aren't putting notes on the board, write the very important notes from your class. Does your history teacher mention dates from different battles? Does your English teacher mention specific parts in Shakespeare's plays? Is your maths teacher going over a certain formula? Write all of these down.

It may take some experimentation to decide which of the information is really useful, so it's good to keep on trying and never give up. Your teachers are going to have different teaching methods. An example would be some of your teachers might mention a lot of facts and dates but only write down the essential facts on their board. Others might not write the things down but they might repeat certain pieces of information or dates. That is a clue that they are likely important. After you have been in their class a while, you are going to learn their teaching style.

Catching important key points your teacher says is crucial and an important part of studying in high school, but don't worry if you miss information.

Do not overdo note taking, trying to write everything down. If you too frantic, trying to write down every word that your teacher says you may miss very important points. Sometimes people learn much better when they are listening, writing a few important points down, and then reading their material when class is done when there's more time.

Ask questions - Never be afraid to ask questions when you are in class. You can ask your teacher if he or she can repeat something if they are going much too fast. Chances are if she is going too fast for you, she's going too fast for other people in the class. If you are not comfortable asking while in class, you can talk with your teacher after class. It's a lot better to ask than wonder if you got the right notes while studying.

Compare your notes - Keep the notes you take handy anytime you're reading your textbooks. Compare the notes you took with the things that are in your books. It may also be a good idea to expound upon on your notes while reading.

Going over the note you have taken with one of your friends who is in the same class as you are and comparing what the two of you have written down can also reinforce the things that you are learning. It can also help with remembering the information when it's time to take your test. Going over the notes is going to help with alerting you and the other person about any kinds of errors.

Copy - If you are taking your notes in a hurry to keep up with your teacher, you are going to have an easier time figuring out something that you can't read when you just took the notes that day than later.

Organize your notes - Mind Maps are a wonderful way to develop your understanding of virtually any topic. You can capture information creatively to boost your productivity and memory.

One great use of Mind Maps is to create them once you get home from school, from the notes you jotted down in your notebook during the lesson. This gives you an opportunity to review everything you learned that day, and organise your ideas properly. If there is anything you don't really   understand from the lesson when creating your Mind Map you now have the chance to look up the point in your textbook for clearer understanding.

The basics of Mind Mapping are:
- Use your paper in landscape format
- Start with a central image to represent your topic
- Use curving lines to add main branches to the centre
- Then connect these to smaller branches; using single words and images
- Add colours for aesthetic and organisational purposes

For further information on Mind Mapping, http://thinkbuzan.com/

Good note-taking will take a lot of additional time and organization. It can help if you think of the time that you spend reviewing your notes as an investment. The time that you take to recopy your notes may mean that you have less time for chatting with your friends or watching television, but you are going to have to study less when you get ready for your test.

Taking notes will give your mind an opportunity to absorb the important material you will need for learning. This will help you do much better on your tests and it will also help boost your confidence while you're studying and you find that it is easier to remember things.

Homework Tips

Homework seems to be the bane of every student's existence. But when you are using the tips below for homework, you will find that it's not as bad as you think it might be.

Create A Plan For Homework

When you have a lot of homework, one of the best things that you can do is to create a plan for your homework. Having a plan will allow you to get everything done in a timely manner. Here are some tips for making your homework into less work.

a. Make sure that you understand your assignment. Write the assignment in your day planner or notebook if it's necessary and never be afraid of asking questions regarding what you have to do. It is a lot easier if you take a moment and ask your teacher during class or after class than struggling to remember when you get home. It's also not a bad idea to ask your teacher how long it will take for you to complete so you're able to budget your homework time.

b. Use extra time that you're given in school for homework time. A lot of schools offer study halls. These are periods specifically for doing homework or studying. It's really tempting to talk with your friends during unstructured time or study periods, but when you are doing more work while in school you won't have as much to do at home.

c. Pace yourself. If you do not do your homework during your school day, consider the amount that's left and the other things that you are doing that day. Having a homework schedule is a great idea, especially if you are involved in activities after school, in sports, or you have a job after school.

d. You need a good homework area – When you're studying or doing your homework, where is it done? Are you doing it while watching television? Are you doing it at the kitchen table while your mother is trying to make dinner and set the table?

That spot might have worked during your elementary school days when you didn't have to concentrate as much on your work. But since you're much older, a study, your bedroom, or another quiet place can be a better idea. But don't sit on your bed to study. First of all, it will relax you. Second of all, you will think of your bed as a place of work and may have trouble sleeping in it. It's better to have a table or desk with a good chair so that you can concentrate and have plenty of room for your books and notebooks.

Start working. When you begin your homework, tackle your most difficult assignments while you're fresh. Even though you might think it's a good idea to do the easy assignments, you want to do the harder ones when you're more focused and energetic.

If you find you're stuck on a certain problem, try your best to do it. At the same time, don't spend a lot of time on it and obsess over it. Doing this can mess up your schedule and make it hard for you to finish. If you have trouble, ask someone to give you some help.

Once you have finished with your homework, look over what you have done to see if you want to make any changes. Then you should place it in a safe place so that you will have it with you the next day.

Tips for Writing a Paper
One of the most common types of homework is writing a paper. It's often intimidating to have to write a paper, particularly if English and writing aren't your favourite subjects. But to put together a very strong paper will just involve different things that you can do already.

Understanding Your Assignment

The first thing to do when you are writing your paper for school is to be sure you understand what the assignment is. Here are a few questions that you should ask before you begin to research and write your paper.

What kind of paper do I need to write? Do I have to write a report where I have to gather the facts, a paper where I have to offer my own opinions on a certain issue, or a combination of both?

Do I have to use certain readings in class as my resources?
What kinds of resources can't I use? Can I only use sources from the Internet, or am I required to use newspapers, journals, and books? Does my teacher want me to conduct interviews or are printed sources the only things I can use?

Are there particular source types that I can't use? Obviously things like personal websites and blogs won't be reliable sources. But can I use other types of websites?

What is my teacher going to look for when she is grading my paper? Is my teacher going to look for a descriptive, casual writing style similar to an article in a magazine or a tone that's more formal such as research papers need? Does my teacher have a certain structure she wants for my paper?
What's the length my paper needs to be in words or pages?

Does my paper need to be done in a particular format or does it have to be typed? Do I have to double space it, put specific margin in it, or present it in a folder or binder? Do I have to include graphics like photos or illustrations?

Do I have to provide footnotes, a bibliography, or other kinds of sources?
Sometimes your teacher is going to assign a thesis or topic for your paper and sometimes she will let you choose the topic. If your teacher allows you to select your own topic, you want to write your

paper about a topic you find interesting. This could be a certain issue about which you feel strongly and you are interested in defending or one that you don't agree with and you want to argue about. After you've come up with a topic, make sure that your teacher is okay with it before starting your research.

Researching Your Topic

Good research helps you write a good paper. When you want to do your research, you mean you have to read a lot, both for background to help you select your topic and then to help you write the paper.

Depending on the topic you select, your research might come from newspapers, websites, professional journals, or even your class text-books. These will be your paper's sources.

The sources you choose have to be reliable. So that you can find reliable sources, start out at the library in your school where the search engines and computers can send you to the published materials. When you choose a source from the collection at your school library, you can be sure that the sources are accurate and good for using on your paper.

Using Online Sources

When you are doing online research, stay away from personal website pages. It will be impossible to know if that person is an expert. You should focus on using government websites, educational websites, and non-profit organizations for your research. These websites domain names end in .gov for government, .edu for educational, and .org for non-profit organizations. Knowing the good and bad sources is one of the skills that you will gain with experience. Ask your librarian and teachers to help you decide on credible sources.

If you do not understand what a certain source is talking about, ask your teacher to explain so you can understand the material better. Teachers are able to tell when a student uses information on their papers they don't truly understand.

Doing your research online when you're doing a project or writing a paper is a great idea. But when you have a lot of choices available to you it can be overwhelming. Knowing the way you can evaluate and select resources online can help you avoid wasting time and headaches.

Here are four ways that you can make your online research as effective and easy as possible.

1. **Begin at school.** Ask your librarian or teacher which resources they are going to recommend for your chosen project. This way you'll be sure that the sources you are using are approved by the school and that their information is accurate. Sometimes, your teacher or school might have paid subscriptions for websites or online journals. These sources can provide you with information you would not get doing regular internet searches.

   Unless you're otherwise told by your teacher, you should use the internet as an additional tool rather than it being your only research tool. The library at school is filled with resources like books and magazines that you can use.

   A lot of schools block the access to entire websites or online images that can be valuable research tools. So you want to make sure that you do research at home, municipal library, or other places where you can get Internet access.

2. **Sort the facts from fiction.** Prior to beginning your research, list the types of websites that are great for researching your topic. You can also use established websites that are news-related, but make sure you are using original sources.
   Sites that end in .org usually are non-profit organizations. These can be good sources for research, but you should check with teachers to be sure that she's happy with the site

and that it's appropriate. Although Wikipedia is very popular, usually it is not a credible source.

On the websites that end in .com, check for advertising. If there's advertising on the website, its thoughts could be biased. Personal websites, social media websites, and blogs may also be biased.

4. **Search wisely**. Begin with an established engine like Bing or Google. You can also use search engines specific to your area.

5. **Remain focused.** When you are prepared to do searches or look at websites, stay off of chat, email, Facebook, and turn your phone off. Stay focused.

When you are doing research online, it can be very easy to copy the text and then paste it, then forget about citing the source. Sometimes you might put those thoughts into your words. Similarly to how teachers are able to recognize your voice when you're in class, your teacher will be able to recognize your style and voice in your writing. Even accidentally plagiarizing can have severe consequences when it comes to grades so you don't want to take a chance. Identify any text you're quoting and add citations before you move on in your paper.

Tracking Your Resources
After you have located a great source, note it so that you are able to use it on your paper. Keep a computer document or notebook that has the title of the source, the important information's page number, and several notes about why this source is important. This is going to help you efficiently move ahead while writing. It will also help you to cite your sources correctly.

Writing The Paper

The best thing about doing a lot of research is that it will help you write your paper since you will really know the topic. But it can also be hard to sit down in front of your computer screen when you know that you have a deadline coming up. Even when you have read a lot of websites, journals, and books, it is common to struggle with getting started.

What is a good way to get started? Simply start putting down your ideas on paper. Those first words don't need to be the best, and chances are they aren't going to be, but you will find it easier once you get started. You will be revising your paper later. The most important thing is to get started. When your ideas are down on paper, you're able to begin outlining them.

Sometimes people think of this attempt as their first draft. This takes pressure off to make it perfect. A second good tip to get started is to jot down the ideas as if you're telling a sister, brother, or parent about them.

Do not feel like the paper has to be written in order. If you're writing a thesis, but you're not sure how it should be introduced, you might write your supporting paragraphs and then write your introduction.

A lot of people make their revisions during their work. An example would be if you're halfway through your fourth paragraph when you come up with a better way to argue the points made in your second paragraph. This is your thinking process and it's why you want to leave a lot of time to do your paper instead of putting the work off until the last minute.

It also is a great idea to give yourself enough time once the paper is finished to it aside and then read it over to see what you want to change. Revising your paper is something that all professional writers think as essential. When you haven't looked at the paper for a period of time, any problems or flaws are going to stand out even more. Look for nonsensical sentences, unnecessary words, and other things that can be awkward.

It also is a good idea to read your paper out loud. Sometimes you are going to notice things when reading it out loud that you didn't notice reading through it.

Citing Sources

Your teacher will want your sources cited, meaning that you are listing your sources for statements, ideas, and any other information in the paper. Make sure that you know how your teacher wants the sources cited.

Citation shows that you have done a lot of research and tells readers where the ideas came from. Citations are not necessary when you are mentioning a commonly known fact, like a battle's date, or when the idea's your own.

Citing your sources is essential because it will help you avoid plagiarism. This is using another person's words or ideas and not giving the person the credit. Students often plagiarize by quoting, copying, or summarizing without citing the spot from which the information came.

Dealing With Stress From Papers

Knowing that you have a paper that needs to be written may be stressful for you. To help avoid getting overwhelmed, these two steps can help.

1. **Begin when it's assigned.** When you do this, you are going to have enough time when something unexpected comes up. This way you have time in case you need extra time for research and if you need to change topics.
2. **Break your paper into mini-projects.** When you have miniature projects, it won't seem as overwhelming. Figure out the amount of time that you need for each of the mini projects. This will help you feel like you're in control and also help you know the amount of time your paper is going to take.

Writing a paper is an exercise in learning and that is the reason why teachers have you do them. Your teachers don't expect perfection, and even college students ask their professors for help. If you find that you need help, you should speak with your teacher.

Study Tips

Even if you don't have a test or quiz coming up, it's always a good idea to study and help yourself remember what you learned in school that day. It will make test days much easier because things can become second nature. Here are some tips that you can use for studying effectively.

Start Your Studying While At School

Studying for quizzes and tests should start long before you know that a test is coming. Your good techniques for studying start in your classroom while you're taking notes. Even though you aren't studying in the usual sense, note-taking is one of the ways you can remember what you have read or you have been taught. Take a look at our section on taking notes to help you.

Plan Your Personal Study Time

Plan how much time you are going to give each of your topics. This will help you from being overwhelmed.

For example, if the day is Monday and you have three tests coming up on Friday, decide the amount of time you'll need to study for the next five days. Then you want to figure out the amount of time each of your subjects is going to take. An example would be if you have a verb test in Spanish every week, it's not likely to be intense compared with a huge history test. That means you won't need as much time to study for your Spanish test as your history test. Break up your topics into smaller chunks to give yourself a good study schedule.

Another technique for studying is called chunking - this breaks large topics into manageable chunks. An example would be if you have a test coming up about WW II. Rather than thinking of studying the whole of WWII, which would be overwhelming to anyone, try breaking the sessions into specific battles or years.

Most people are able to concentrate for approximately 45 minutes well. After that you will likely want to take a brief break. If you are finding that you're becoming distracted with your mind drifting to other things while you're studying, make sure you're pulling your thoughts back to your studying. Keep in mind that every 45 minutes worth of studying is equal to 15 minutes of break.

Breaks are essential to maximise the greatest harmony between recall, understanding and mental fatigue. Short breaks, of course will give you chance to chat with your friend, but importantly, will help you limit muscular and mental tension which always cause strain on your body when concentrating on your studying.

Do your studying based on your kind of test

A lot of teachers let students know ahead of time the exam format that they will be taking. This will help to plan the way that you are studying. If the teacher says it will be a multiple-choice test, you will want to put your focus on details and facts. But if it's going to be an essay test, you will want to consider the topics which the test will likely cover. Then you want to think of three possible topics and then use your books, notes, and other types of reference sources so that you can figure out the way you may answer the questions about those topics.

As you are studying, review the notes and any kind special information your textbook contains. Read important facts over a few times if necessary, and write down thoughts or phrases that are going to help you remember the main concepts or ideas.

When you're trying to remember names, dates, or other kinds of factual information, remember that it takes a few tries before you're able to correctly remember something. That's one of the reasons why it is smart to begin studying long before the night before a test. Use special triggers to help your memory that your teacher suggested or even that you came up with yourself.

When it comes to science or math equations or problems, practice various problems. Give special attention to the things that your teacher stresses during class.

Sometimes people find that it's helpful to teach imaginary students what they are studying. It also can be helpful to choose someone to study with and then teach each other. Another technique for studying is to make flashcards which summarize different concepts or facts. They can be used for reviewing for tests.

Don't Procrastinate

It's really tempting to put off your studying right until the night before the test. But you won't do well on the test like this. So you want to make sure that you are studying from the time you are given the work.

If you like procrastinating, a good way to overcome this problem is to stay organized. Once you have written down dates when projects are due and when you will be taking tests, it's really hard to forget them. When you sit down to plan and organize your work, it will really highlight the amount of time it will take. When you are organized, you will find it's harder for you to procrastinate.

Sometimes you will put off studying because you feel overwhelmed and that that you're behind on other work or you're really feeling disorganized. This is something you want to avoid. Keep all of your notes well organized, make sure you're staying on top of the things you need to read, and follow all of the tips that are mentioned here for staying in control and focused. You will get a lot of notice regarding important tests so you have plenty of time to study for the different exams you are taking.

Sometimes you might feel overwhelmed because of activities outside of regular classes. Ask for help prioritizing your schedule from your teachers. It may be that you'll need involvement from coaches or music and drama teachers so that a solution can be worked out.

Do not wait until the last minute to speak with your teachers, or you are going to look like you're a procrastinator. Never feel afraid to request help. Your teachers are going to respect you for being thoughtful and showing interest in the learning process and performing well in school.

Begin Study Groups

Often it's useful to review what you are studying with other people from your group. You can be sure that the notes you took are right and that you understand the topic. Study groups are also helpful since you're able to work with one another to think of ways to remember concepts before testing each other.

However, if you are someone who gets distracted easily, a study group can be a bad idea since they often get off-topic. When you are with a group of classmates or friends, you might spend more time gossiping than you do studying. One of the ways that you can ensure focus and quiet when you're studying as a group is to go to the library. You are going to be forced to keep the topics and discussions quieter than when you are at a friend's house.

The Payoff

Once you're done studying, you ought to feel as if you're able to approach your quiz or test confidently. This doesn't mean that you are going to ace the test, but you are going to have a better understanding of that information.

Lastly, do not panic if you're unable to remember some of the facts the evening before your test. Even when you have spent the whole night studying, your brain will need time to digest the information. You will be surprised at the things you remember after you have had a good night's sleep.

Test Taking Tips

Tests are a fact of school life and are important to show your teacher what you have learned. But it's normal to feel a bit stressed out when it comes to taking a test. In fact, there are times when a bit of adrenaline (a hormone that's made inside your body when you are excited or stressed out) will help you perform at your best.

Here are a few general tips when taking tests:

- **Make sure you properly studied.** This sounds like it should be a given, but if you are certain about the test information, you are going to feel less stressed out.

- **Get a good night's sleep.** This is the biggest mistakes my students often make. Your ability to recall information is going to be a lot better if you have had ample rest. A study showed that the people who got enough sleep before they took a test got better scores than the people who spent the whole night before cramming.

- **Listen to the instructions carefully**. As your teacher is handing out the tests, make sure you are aware of what you have to do.

- **Read through your test.** Once you've received your test paper, read over your whole test, checking the length of it and the parts you need to complete. This is going to let you estimate the amount of time you'll have for each of the sections. If something appears unclear, ask about it at the beginning.

- **Focus on each of the questions individually.** As you're taking your test, if you aren't' sure of one of the answers, don't become obsessed. Either answer it the best you can or skip it and then go back to the question once you've answered the others.

- **Relax.** Relaxation is important. When you're a nervous wreck, it may be that you need a tiny break. Of course, you aren't able to stand up and walk around during a test, but you're able to wiggle your toes and fingers, take a few deep breaths, or use imaging to take you to a calm place like a beach.

- **Go over the answers.** If you finish early, it is a good idea to go over your answers. You also may be able to add some more details that you didn't think of before.

The above tips can be used for just about any type of tests. Now that I have given you some tips on some general test taking, I am going to give you some more specific tips that cover different types of tests.

Essay Test Taking Tips
Essay tests are often one of the most feared types of tests that students take. But if you know the way to take them, they do not have to be as worrisome. Here are some of the tips that you can use for taking essay tests.

- Carefully read your directions. Make sure you read how many essays you are supposed to answer.
- Be sure you understand the questions. If you aren't sure, ask the teacher.
- Be sure that you are answering the question properly. When you provide a lot of facts and details, you are going to get a higher grade.
- Be sure you budget your time. Be sure you do not devote your whole amount of time on a single essay. If you are given an hour to write three essays, don't spend in excess of 20 minutes per essay.
- Try to write neatly which will generally receive a higher mark.
- Create an outline prior to writing an essay. Because of this, you will have an essay that's more fluid and organized. If don't finish before the test is over, most teachers will give you some credit before your ideas in your outline.
- Do not write lengthy introductions & conclusions. Most of your time needs to be spent on the question that has been asked.
- Focus on a single idea per paragraph.

- If there's time when you have finished, proof read what you have written and fix any of your errors.

True or False Test Taking Tips

True and false tests are a favourite of many students since they know they have a 50/50 chance of getting the right answer. Here are some tips that you can use to have a better chance of getting a good score on your next true or false test.

- Generally there will be more answers that are true rather than answers that are false.
- If there isn't a guessing penalty, you should guess. You will have a 50% chance to get the correct answer.
- Read through the statements carefully, and give close attention to keywords and qualifiers.
- Qualifiers such as "always, every, and never" mean the statement has to be true constantly. Generally these kinds of qualifiers will mean it's false.
- Qualifiers like sometimes, generally, and usually mean the statement is able to be considered false or true based on certain circumstances. Generally these qualifiers mean that the answer is true.
- If any of the question is false, the whole statement will be false. However, simply because a statement is partially true doesn't make the whole statement true.

Tips for Multiple Choice Tests

Multiple choice tests are another type of test that many students look forward to since they know that the right answer is there. They just have to choose it. Here are some tips for taking multiple choice tests.

- Read the question completely before you look at your choices.
- Answer the question before you look at your possible answers. This will help you from being swayed by the wrong answers.
- Eliminate any answer you know is incorrect.

- Read all of your choices before you select your answer.
- If there isn't a guessing penalty, take educated guesses and choose your answer.
- Don't keep changing answers. Generally the first choice will be the correct one. This doesn't apply, of course, if you read your question wrong.
- In choices that read All or None, if you're sure that one of your choices is right, then don't choose "None." If one of your choices is false, don't choose "All."
- If the question has an "All" choice, if you see a minimum of two right statements, then the answer probably is "All".
- Positive choices are usually truer than negative ones.
- Generally the right answer is the one that has the most amount of information.

Oral Test Taking Tips

Oral exams aren't as common as other types of tests, but they are sometimes done. If you have an oral exam coming up, here are some of the tips that you can use when you're facing one.

- Confirm the place and time of the test with the teacher.
- Find out the topics you are going to be tested upon, and if you're permitted to bring visual aids, props, and the way to dress.
- Prepare for your oral exam like you would another exam.
- Anticipate any questions the exam might have. Prepare the answers for those questions and then ask and answer the questions you believe you may be asked using another person. If possible, the person should be somebody in your class who's familiar with the material.
- Practice speaking before a mirror so you're able to evaluate the language of your body. Another thing you can do is to record the answers you give and then play them back so you're able to listen to the way you sound. If possible, have someone use their phone to make a video so you can see your composure and the way you sound.

- If you're using equipment such as a computer for the exam, test it a few times to make certain everything is how you would like it to be.
- Arrive at your exam a few minutes before it starts so you don't feel rushed. If you are late, it could negatively impact your grade.
- Turn your mobile phone off before you take your exam.
- Dress appropriately.
- Maintain good posture and eye contact. Do not slouch if you are sitting down and don't lean if you are standing.
- Give the questions close attention. If you do not understand a question, ask your examiner to clarify it or ask for the question to be repeated.
- Your answers should be given in sentences that are complete. If it's possible, don't give answers of one or two words.
- Make sure that you thank your instructor for their time when the test is over.

Tips for Taking Short Answer Tests

Short answer tests are tests in which there are no options but the answers don't have to be as long as an essay question. Here are some tips for taking short answer tests.

- Create flashcards. Put the key dates, concepts, and terms on the front of the cards and the events, explanations, and definitions on the back.
- Try anticipating the questions which are going to be asked on your test and get ready for them. Generally the things that are emphasized in class are going to be on tests.
- If possible, don't leave any answers blank. Write down your thoughts and show your working out. Even if the answer isn't exact, you may be given partial credit.
- If you do not know an answer, leave it alone and then go back once the test is finished. Make a guess. Other test questions might provide clues to the answer.

- Read the questions carefully and be sure you answer all parts. Some of the questions on short answer tests will have more than one part.

Tips for Taking Open Book Tests

Contrary to popular belief, open book tests are not as easy as they may seem. They require as much, if not more, thought than tests in which a book cannot be used.

- Spend the same amount of time or even more getting ready for an open book test as you would for a regular test. Open book exams are often much harder than close book exams.
- Become familiar with your book and the relevant materials.
- If you're allowed, jot down the key information and important formulas on another sheet before you start.
- Focus upon learning your main ideas. Get a good idea of where they're found in your book. If there is extra time, learn the other details later.
- Use bookmarks, highlight the important points, use sticky notes, and make some notes inside your book if you can.
- Bring all of the resources you are permitted to bring.
- Answer the easy questions first that you can without looking them up and then do the harder questions where you will have to look up the answers.
- Use some quotations from your book in order to support the view you have, but do not over-quote. Make sure that you give your own commentary and insight.

Tips for Taking Quantitative/Math Tests

For many people, maths is their worst subject. But if you know how to prepare properly, they don't have to be so frightening. Here are some tips for taking math tests.

- Repetition is essential in maths. You learn the way to solve problems when you keep doing them, so keep doing practice problems. However, don't do them blindly. Be sure you learn the way to recognize why/when you need to use specific methods to solve problems.

- Work on some practice problems by topic, ranging in difficulty levels.
- When you are practicing, try solving problems by yourself, then look at the answers or ask for help if you have trouble.
- Mix up the order of the questions from the different topics when you're reviewing so that you will learn when specific formulas/methods need to be used.
- Create a sheet with the necessary formulas and then memorize the formulas that are on your sheet.
- When you receive your exam, jot down your key formulas in the margin at the beginning.
- Carefully read your directions and do not forget that all parts of your question need to be answered.
- Show your working out, particularly when you will be awarded partial credit. Make sure that you are writing legibly.
- If you know your final answer is wrong, you shouldn't erase your work since you could receive partial credit since you used the right procedure.
- Look at your test once you are done. If there's enough time, redo your problems on another paper to see if you're getting the same answers. Look for any careless mistakes like making sure your decimal points are in the correct place, that you have read your directions right, that the numbers were copied correctly, and that you have placed the negative sign if it's needed.

Responsibility Around The House

Responsibility is so important in all aspects of your life. Now that you are older, it is very important that you help your parents out more around the house. This means taking on some of the chores around the house.

Here are some of the chores that you should be doing around the house now that you are a teenager. Honestly, by the time you are a teenager, you should be capable to handle almost any household task. My sister and I were doing every chore listed below by the time we were 8 and 9, so nothing is beyond a teenager.

Teenagers should not expect their parents to do everything for them. You should keep your room clean and neat, leave the bathroom in good order, and pick up after yourself as an absolute minimum.

Do not ever think you are too busy to take care of your personal responsibilities. Just because you are doing well at school, got lots of activities to do outside of school, or even got a part-time job, it does not mean you can relieve yourself of your chores.

Taking care of household chores will prepare you very well for when you are older. You will be training your mind and body to develop beneficial life habits, which will prepare you so well for the future.

Being a good family citizen is a very special value to have, so don't wait for your parents to ask you to help them out around the home – just start off your own back!

Vacuuming
- Vacuum all room and stairs
- Furniture
- Change the bag in the vacuum cleaner when applicable
- Sweeping
- Kitchen and Bathroom floors

Laundry
- Gather up dirty clothes and dirty towels from bathroom
- Put laundry into washer, put clean clothes into the dryer
- Fold and put away clean laundry
- Wipe off dryer and washer

Dusting
- Dust all top surfaces in every room around the house
- Ceiling fans, blinds and Computer desk

General Cleaning

- Tidy up family room and living room, and use lint brush on any furniture
- Wipe down living room baseboards / skirting boards in every room
- Wipe down light switches and doorknobs
- Collect rubbish from different rooms
- Clean computer screen and keyboard
- Walk the dog/clean out any litter trays
- Water any plants
- Wash tile floors in bathroom/kitchen
- Shake the dust off any rugs outside
- Wash the car, clean and vacuum the inside

Kitchen Chores

- Clean cabinets and counters
- Wash dishes/load and unload dishwasher
- Make dinner (parents should leave instructions)
- Make lunches for yourself and siblings
- Set and clear the table
- Give water and feed pets
- Clean door and shelves of fridge, interior and exterior
- Remove old food from fridge
- Clean toaster, unplugging it and dumping out the crumbs

Window washing

- Wash all windows in every room
- Stairwell or hallway
- Chores in the Spring and Summer
- Mow and trim the lawn
- Trim bushes

- Weed garden
- Clean outdoor furniture
- Remove outdoor furniture from storage and wipe them down
- Care for pool and vacuum it
- Take care of siblings while they're out of school

Chores in the Autumn
- Rake and bag leaves
- Clean outside furniture and store for the winter

Chores in the Winter
- Shovel snow
- Clean snow from car
- Get car washed to get rid of salt
- Help with holiday decorations

Babysitting

Since we listed caring for younger siblings in the chores that you should do, we decided that it would be best to go over some of the things that are important to know when you are responsible for children. These tips apply whether you are looking after your siblings or someone has hired you to babysit their children.

Before we even get into babysitting and the things that you should do to make sure that your charges are safe, let's go over 3 very important things that you need to know.

How to Contact Parents
Make sure that before you start looking after the children that you have the right numbers and information. This has gotten a little bit easier since most parents have cell phones now, but they still need to have the phone on so you can get in touch with them.

Where Are The Medical Supplies and Information

If you are watching your own siblings, you should know where this is. But if you are watching someone else's children, you will need this information.   Make sure that you know the allergies, medications, health issues, and anything else that you need to know about the children.

A parent should have a kit that has things like plasters, antibacterial cream, and alcohol wipes in it handy.   Know where it's kept, what's kept in the kit, and how the items should be used. If you need to use something from the kit, tell the parents so that they can restock the items.

You also need to know what can be used on the kids and what can't. a lot of kits have pain medicines in them, but not all of them can be used on children. Always ask what the children can take and what they can't.

If a child needs to be given medication while you are watching them, you should be shown how to do it. Check the expiration of the medicine before giving it.   Close the bottles tightly once you have measured the right dose.

Sometimes a child has an allergy that is bad enough to require injections. If the child you are watching has one, know where the auto-injector is and the way to use it.

How to Keep Them Safe

Kids love exploring and they often will quickly find trouble. Accidents happen and sometimes the accident requires a doctor or hospital visit. That's why you have to constantly supervise them. Make sure that you are always watching them, particularly around heaters, appliances, water, and other kinds of hazards.   Keep any medications out of kids' reach.

If the parents ask you to do something you didn't do before, ask them to let you know the way they want it done. If they want you to take them somewhere in a car, for example, it's essential to know the car seats that are to be used and the proper way for them to be buckled in. Ask that they demonstrate it for you. You can also ask if you can use their car since it's easier and safer if you're using a seat that's installed already.

Know where the parents keep their emergency and safety equipment, such as flashlights, batteries, and fire extinguishers. Emergencies mean that you have to have the right equipment but it also is important to know where it is, how it's to be used, and what to do.

Before Your Babysitting Job

- Get information from parents, including address, the number of children, the ages and names of children, and any medical conditions.
- Agree upon the hours you'll be working, your rate, and what you need to do. If you're not sure about pay rate, check with people who have done babysitting or get advice from your parents.
- Meet children and parents before beginning so you are able to become familiar with one another before the time you meet.
- Know the numbers for emergency.
- Prepare activities for the kids. Be sure that you are preparing weather suitable, safe, and fun for everyone.
- Tell your parents where you're going to be and when you'll be home or when they need to get you.

During Your Babysitting Job

- When you get to the house for your first job, ask that they show you the house so you understand the layout. Do not be afraid if you have any questions – when you know a lot, you are going to do a better job.
- Before they leave, be sure you're comfortable with the rules of the house, how they discipline children, and their expectations of you. If you aren't sure about something, ask.

- When you are babysitting, never leave the children alone. Keep an eye out for any hazards in the home like toys on stairs, unclosed gates, appliances that are left on, or any small items that children might grab and choke on. You should never assume that it's going to be fine.

- Follow the rules. Never invite any rules over and don't use their internet or phone unless you have been told you're allowed to.

- Respect the differences and know that families often have other ways to do things.

- Clean up. Try leaving the house like it was when you came.

- Remain calm in an emergency. Call the emergency number and follow any advice you receive from the emergency services.

- When the children's parents come back, let them know about any problems you had. You want to be up front regarding problems instead of having them find out.

- When you return home, tell your own parents about anything that made you feel worried or uncomfortable during your babysitting job.

Chapter 9
The Best For Last: Love & Dating

Now that you are a teenager, you will be more and more excited about going out on a date. Actually chances are that you have been excited about doing it before now, but you were just too young. You are going into a whole new world with new things to discover and new fears to overcome.

Love can be one of the scariest things that you will ever experience. When you are in love, you will often experience tremendous highs and lows. You are going to have some of the strongest feelings you have ever had in your life. This is awesome when they are good feelings. But when things aren't so good, they can make you devastated. Below are 7 tips that you can use to help things go well during this exciting and confusing time.

Dating Tip 1: Go Slow
Some teenagers date and some don't. According to Charles Wibbelsman of Kaiser Permanente, an adolescent specialist and pediatrician in San Francisco, it's important for you to feel good about yourself before you start dating. You should only date if you're ready to date and you know all about yourself. You shouldn't date because everyone else is dating.

Dating Tip 2: Find a Person Who Likes You
When your feelings aren't returned, this can make you question a lot of things about yourself. Was it something you said? Did you wear the wrong thing? In healthy relationships, people are mutually attracted. You're respecting one another and you're having fun with one another. If this isn't your situation, there isn't anything wrong personally with you. You simply need to keep on looking.

Dating Tip 3: Know When It's Time for You to Move On

There are times when you know that the relationship just isn't working. Maybe the person that you love has turned out to be selfish and mean. Maybe you realize you want something that's better. According to Danielle Greaves, who counsels girls in Massachusetts, it's essential to find someone who will give you the things you need. It's going to hurt, but you'll get through it.

Dating Tip 4: Don't Put Everything on Facebook

If you have a boyfriend, chances are you want to let the whole world know. But it's not necessary to put it on Facebook. Keep some things just between the two of you. The last thing that you need is a lot of pressure from other people. Also remember there are dangerous predators on the Internet, so please value your privacy.

Dating Tip 5: Guard Yourself Against Pressure

Pressure isn't love and it's not normal. Chances are that you aren't going to face any pressure from someone that you are dating. But in case that you are, it's best to be ready to give your answers. Figure out what you value and the furthest you're ready to go. If you do this, you will not have to decide when and if the moment comes.

Here are a couple of things to make sure you stay out of a personal pressure chamber:

- Stay away from the situations in which a guy may expect something more than you're ready to give.
- Date the guys who are near your own age. The girls who date guys who are older are much more likely to become to be rushed into being sexually active before they are ready.

Dating Tip 6: Give Your Love Time for It to Grow

A lot of times the thought of love's much better than the real thing. How are you going to know if you really truly are in love?

174

If you are infatuated, you are looking for constant reassurance, and you can't think about other things, you probably aren't in love. It's a lot of fun but you are probably going to feel disappointed eventually. Love that's mature will grow stronger as time goes on. As you are getting to know one another, you will have stronger feelings. If it's true love, you won't have to be somebody you aren't. You like the other person for themselves and they are the same with you. If you are like most people, this is going to take a while to find this mature love. The good news is that it's worth it to be patient in the end.

Dating Tip 7: Never Put Dating Before Studying

One of the biggest mistakes I hear most often is from people who thought their teen relationship was the most important thing in the world at that time. They let that relationship damage their studying, only to see the relationship fizzle out later, and they were left is very difficult situations to try and repair the damage done to their education.

Question 1. Are you ready to date?

When most girls are asked whether or not they are ready to start dating, they will say YES without a second thought. But are you REALLY? Have you thought about all of the things that go with dating, the good and the bad? Sure, dating means that you are going out with someone and that you have a date to dances. But it also can mean heartbreak. Let's look at some of the things that dating can mean.

- **Loss of personal space**. Until now, you have had a lot of personal space. Dating means that you are going to be holding hands, kissing, hugging, and possibly doing other things with another person.
- **Pressure.** Although you'd like to think that every person you date is going to be willing to wait until you're ready for sex, that's often not the case. Do you know what you are going to do in that situation?

- **Emotional and Physical Rejection**. Are you going to be ready for rejection from someone that you loved? Whenever you open up to another person, physically or emotionally, and you find yourself rejected, you are going to feel hurt.
- **Dumping Someone**. Dumping works both ways. What happens if you find that you aren't happy in your relationship? Are you ready and mature enough to break it off? Could you be kind but firm at the same time and do it?

Your readiness to date should never be based on everyone else. Even when it appears as if everyone's dating, you shouldn't date for the heck of it. You should date someone because you like them, not because you are feeling left out since everyone else has a boyfriend/girlfriend.

A good example of this is the episode on Full House in which Stephanie is invited to a make-out party and she's uncomfortable. So she calls her dad. You should never do anything because everyone else is doing it. You should do what's right for you.

Question 2. Do you truly like the person?

Now you should think about the person that you like. Why is it that you really like them? Do you like them because they are really good looking? If that's the case, it's not the right reason.

When you are interested in someone, you have to share common interests. You will also want to be with a person who is going to treat you the right way.

How will you be able to tell? One of the best clues is the way they're treating their teachers, friends, and parents.

If you aren't completely sure about the person, ask yourself if it is even worth starting a relationship. You can also ask your friends and get their input whether or not they are worth it.

Question 3. Is the Person the Right One for You?

One of the most important questions to ask is whether the person's safe for dating.

If you want to date older guys, you should be very careful. Dating a guy who is much older than you are can be dangerous. If you're in middle school and you like a guy who's in high school or you're a freshman and you want to date a senior, you may find yourself pressured into doing something you don't want to do.

Just because you might look older it doesn't mean that you're ready for dating older boys. Boys who are older tend to have more experience and may expect more from the girls they are dating, according to Laura Choate, who is a licensed counsellor and who wrote Girls' and Women's Wellness: Contemporary Counselling Issues and Interventions.

There was a study done which discovered that girls who were freshmen in high school and who dated guys who were in their junior or their senior year often went further and they were also forced into doing things they weren't ready for or didn't want to do.

It's a good idea to stay away from dating someone who is more than a grade higher than you. Perhaps just resist the temptation to date a guy quite a bit older than you. You could save yourself a lot of stress and disappointment.

Question 4. Are My Parents Going to Let Me Date?

This is the biggest question, since if they say no, you won't get really far. They may say no because they're really conservative, or they are remembering the way they were acting as teens. No matter what the reason is, your parents may tell you no until you are a particular age. Depending on your parents, this age could be 13 or 14, but it also could be up to age 18.

If you truly want to date and your parents aren't giving in, try speaking with them. Do not be confrontational. Be conversational.

You should never say things like "You're mean! All my friends are dating!" If you act like a child, chances are that they aren't going to bend.

It's a good idea to show your parents that you are mature and you're responsible. Remind your parents about the way you're doing in school (if you're doing well in school) and the chores you are doing. Tell them why you really like this person and why you are interested in going out on a date. Even though you might think the person is really good looking, it's probably not a good idea to tell them that as a reason.

A good way to show your parents how this will work is to have a compromise. Maybe see if you can get together with some friends and your guy with your parents' supervision. Then maybe some couple time, but still when you're around your parents. You have to ease them into it.

As time goes by, you will be able to ask for more time alone with your boyfriend, proving that you're mature enough to handle the freedom.

When You Begin Dating

After it's decided that you're ready to start dating and that they are comfortable with the person you're dating, you will be able to begin going out. But when you're starting any type of new relationship, make sure you're taking it slow.

Don't be alone with them completely until you get to know them better. The truth is that abuse is a lot more common in teen dating than you may think. Based on studies by the *Centers for Disease Control and Prevention (CDC)*, 1 in 4 teens has been physically, emotionally, sexually, or verbally abused by someone they're dating.

Whenever someone you are dating forces you into something, demeans you, or strikes you, make sure that you immediately leave the relationship and tell an adult that you trust.

Finally, you should never become so wrapped up in someone you're dating that you are forgetting yourself. If you dress sexy so that you are impressing the person you're dating or you are acting in a way that isn't normal for you, you're losing yourself.

Keep in mind that you are the person that's most important, not the person you are dating. Be true to yourself, and your parents. Don't do anything you think your parents will not be proud of.

The no.1 rule in dating as a teenager is that there is no rush, and however important you think your relationship is right now, it will most likely not mean that much in a few months from now.

Greg & Cristina Noland

Chapter 10
OMG Final Words

When I was a teenager I often felt confused and stressed. I vehemently desired to have a career in sports. When I thought that wasn't going to happen, I looked at what possible career could give me happiness. When a profession didn't jump out at me, I felt even more anxiety. I then looked to my school for guidance but regrettably I never attended a school that pushed its students for higher excellence.

It was at this point of confusion when one of my uncles gave me some life changing advice. "Don't restrict your life by marrying someone with the same passport as you, the world has an abundance of opportunities waiting for you."

It was then that I stopped stressing out thinking about my life and future. I realized that the world is a huge place, and that I needed to relax and give life a chance to show me what it had in store for me.

There is no need for a teenager to feel insecure, inadequate, inferior, or useless. You are only a teenager once, so try your best to enjoy yourself.

Don't blame other people around you for everything that might not be perfect your life.
Don't feel anger for the financial position you feel you are in
Don't feel anger for things that happened when you were young.

Healthy Mind – Body & Spirit Action Guide

Empower yourself to create something different from this moment forward.

- Start a yoga class or get yourself a yoga mat and follow some yoga sessions on Youtube.

- Spend some quality time working out your goals in life.
- Start your Morning Rituals.

Use mine as a start, but feel free to blend your own ideas into your own rituals which you feel confident doing every morning. Promise me that you will try them for 60 straight days,
Please email Cristina or myself, we'd be happy to hear from you.

Please always know you can email me and tell me how you feel about this book.

Please email me at greg@omgteenbookseries.com or Cristina on cristina@omgteenbookseries.com with your feedback about anything you have read in this book, or any of the other books in the **OMG Teen Book Series.**

Being a teenage girl is a very difficult time and you have a lot on your mind. We hope that you have found our book very informative and interesting, and that it has answered a lot of your questions.
Please remember there will be times when you feel strong, and others when you will feel life sucks. Sometimes you will feel supreme confidence, and other times a little insecure or depressed.
This is what it means to be human in this huge and wide-open world. This is life.
We will inevitably experience hurt in our lives, but we don't have to frequently beat ourselves up about it. I hope this book helps you see and treat yourself differently—and live life differently as a result.
We will have many more books coming out in the near future that we are sure that you will find very helpful.
Please keep an eye out for many more books coming out just for you!

Oh, and, Thank You Uncle Emil…

Glossary of Terms

Abstinence

Not having sex of any kind.

Addiction

Needing physical things, such as drugs or alcohol, or an activity, such as stealing or lying, to the point that stopping it is very hard. Stopping can also cause bad physical and mental re-actions. Addiction can be treated with counselling, which means talking to an expert. In some cases, medicine is needed.

Aerobic

Exercise that burns fat, gets your heart rate going, and makes your heart muscle stronger. It helps your blood carry more needed oxygen to blood vessels throughout your body.

AIDS

A disease that hurts the immune system, the body's way of protecting itself. Having AIDS makes it easy to get certain infections and cancers. It is caused by the HIV infection.

Alcoholism

Drinking a lot of alcohol and needing alcohol. Also called alcohol abuse, this disease can lead to injury, liver disease, and problems with the people around you.

Anaerobic

Exercise that builds muscle strength in different parts of your body. This type of exercise goes along well with aerobic exercise. Stronger muscles help you to burn more calories.

Astringents

A product that cleans the skin and tightens the pores.

Birth Control

Prevention of pregnancy.

Cancer

When cells that are not normal grow and can spread. There are at least 200 different kinds of cancers, which can grow in almost any organ of the body.

Cervix

The lower, narrow end of the uterus, which protrudes into the vagina. The muscles of the cervix are flexible so that it can expand to let a baby pass through during birth.

Clitoris

A sensitive female sexual organ that can become erect. The clitoris is part of the vulva.

Condom

A thin sheath used to cover the penis during sex to prevent sexually transmitted diseases and pregnancy.

Douche/douching

Rinsing or cleaning out the vagina, usually with a fluid mix you can buy. The liquid is held in a bottle and squirted into the vagina through tubing and a nozzle. Doctors do not suggest douching to clean the vagina. It changes the chemical balance in the vagina, which can make you more likely to get infections.

Emphysema

A disease that damages the air sacs in the lungs. The air sacs have trouble deflating once filled with air, so they are unable to fill up again with the fresh air you need. Cigarette smoking is the most common cause of emphysema.

Endometrium

The lining of the uterus.

Fallopian tube

Organs that connect the ovaries to the uterus. There is a fallopian tube on each side of the uterus. When one of the ovaries lets go of an egg, it travels through the fallopian tube toward the uterus. Fertilization (when a man's sperm and a woman's egg join together) usually happens in the fallopian tube.

Heart disease

Coronary artery disease, the most common type of heart disease, happens when the heart doesn't get enough blood. Other types of heart disease involve the heart muscle and blood vessels.

Herpes simplex virus

A common virus that has two types: type 1 (HSV-1) and type 2 (HSV-2). Herpes on the mouth shows up as cold sores or fever blisters. This type is mostly caused by HSV-1. Herpes in the genital area is mostly caused by HSV-2, also causing sores. But, both types can affect either the genital area or the mouth.

Hymen

A piece of tissue that covers all or part of the entrance to the vagina. This tissue can be broken the first time a woman has sexual intercourse.

Immunizations

These keep people from getting sick by protecting the body against certain diseases. Also called vaccines, they have parts or products of infectious germs that have been changed or killed. A vaccine gets the body's immune system ready to fight off that germ. Most immunizations that stop you from catching diseases like measles, whooping cough, and chicken pox are given by a shot.

Infertility

When a couple has problems getting pregnant after one year of regular sexual intercourse without using any types of birth control. Infertility can be caused by a problem with the man or the woman, or both.

Labia

The folds of tissue that make up part of the outside female genital area. There are both inner and outer labia.

Lymph glands

A group of cells that make and send out other cells that fight infection throughout the body. These cells help filter out bacteria. Lymph glands are also called lymph nodes.

Menstrual Period

The discharge of blood and tissue from the uterus that occurs when an egg is not fertilized (also called menstruation, period).

Mons pubis

The fatty tissue that covers the pubic area in women. During puberty, hair grows on this area.

Nonacnegenic

Makeup or skin products that should not cause acne.

Noncomedogenic

Makeup or skin products that should not clog pores.

Nutrient

A source of energy, mainly a part of food.

Obstetrician/Gynaecologist (ob-gyn)

A physician with special skills, training, and education in women's health.

Osteoporosis

A disease that causes bones to become thinner and weaker. This disease causes bones to break easily.

Ovary/ovaries

Two small organs on each side of the uterus, in the pelvis of a female. The ovaries have eggs (ova) and make female hormones. When one of the ovaries lets go of an egg about once each month as part of the menstrual cycle, it is called ovulation.

Pads

Sanitary products that stick to the inside of underwear and soak up the blood that leaves the vagina during a menstrual period.

Pap Test

A test in which cells are taken from the cervix and vagina and examined under a microscope.

Pelvic Exam

A manual examination of a woman's reproductive organs.

Pelvic inflammatory disease (PID)

A general term for infection of the lining of the uterus, fallopian tubes, or the ovaries. PID is mostly caused by bacteria that causes STDs, such as chlamydia and gonorrhoea. The most common symptoms include abnormal vaginal discharge (fluid), lower stomach pain, and sometimes fever.

Premenstrual syndrome (PMS)

A group of symptoms that start around 7 to 14 days before the period begins. There are many symptoms, including tender breasts and mood swings. Women may have none, some, or many PMS symptoms. Some months may be worse than others.

Pubic

The area on and around the genitals.

Rectum

The last part of the digestive tract, from the colon to the anus. This is where faeces is stored before leaving the body.

Reproductive

This body system is in charge of making a baby. In women, the body parts involved arc the uterus, ovaries, fallopian tubes, and vagina.

Sexually Transmitted Diseases (STDs)

Diseases that are spread by sexual contact.

Speculum

An instrument used to hold open the walls of the vagina.

SPF

Stands for sun protection factor rating system. Dermatologists advise that SPF 15 or higher sunscreen should be worn every day.

Tampons

These go inside the vagina to soak up blood before it leaves the vagina during a menstrual period. Instructions come with tampon products to show how to use them.

Toxic shock syndrome (TSS)

A very rare but dangerous illness that affects the whole body. TSS is caused by bacteria that make toxins (poisons) in the body. Tampon use can make it easier for bacteria to enter the body. Signs include high fever that comes on suddenly, dizziness, rash, and feeling confused.

Type 2 diabetes

People with diabetes have problems changing food into energy. The body makes insulin to help change glucose (sugar) into energy. Type 2 diabetes usually starts with the muscle, liver, and fat cells not using insulin in the right way. The body tries to make more insulin to meet the demand, but in time, it isn't able to make enough.

Uterus

A pear-shaped, hollow organ in a female's pelvis where a baby grows during pregnancy. It is also called a womb. The uterus is made up of muscle with an inside lining called the endometrium. This lining builds up and thickens during the menstrual cycle to get ready for a possible pregnancy each month. If no pregnancy happens, the extra tissue and blood are shed during menstruation.

UVA

A type of ultraviolet light which that can harm the skin. UVA rays can reach deep into the skin and cause damage. Broad spectrum sunscreens can block both UVA and UVB rays.

UVB

A type of ultraviolet light which can harm the skin. UVB rays are most often the cause of sunburns you can see. Broad-spectrum sunscreens can block both UVA and UVB rays.

Vagina

A muscular tube-like passage that leads down from the cervix, the lower part of the uterus, to the outside of a female's body. During menstruation, menstrual blood flows from the uterus through the cervix and out of the body through the vagina. The vagina is also called the birth canal.

Vaginal discharge

This fluid cleans the vagina and keeps it moist to help fight infections. The colour, amount, and the way it feels will vary during the menstrual cycle. The fluids should be clear, white, or off-white. Discharge that has a foul odour, a change in colour, or a change in how it feels should be checked out by a doctor or at a clinic.

Vulva

The external female genital area which covers the entrance to the vagina and has five parts: mons pubis, labia, clitoris, urinary tract opening, and vaginal opening.

Warts

Genital warts in women are found near or on the vulva, vagina, cervix, or anus. They look like bumps or growths that can be flat or raised, alone or in groups, and big or small. These warts are caused by HPV or human papillomavirus, which is passed by sexual contact.

Yeast infections

A common infection in women caused by an overgrowth of the fungus Candida. It is normal to have some yeast in the vagina, but sometimes it can overgrow during pregnancy or because of taking certain medicines, such as antibiotics. Symptoms include itching, burning, and irritation of the vagina. There may also be pain when urinating and vaginal discharge that looks like cottage cheese.

About The Authors

Greg Noland is the CEO & Founder of The Bum Gun Company. He is an entrepreneur, internet marketer, author, life coach, health & fitness enthusiast, and when he can find the time, a world traveller. Greg started his first business at the age of 9, and had a team of 4 employees before his eleventh birthday, and just grown since then.

Greg is the author of *The Book On The Bum Gun – The Secrets to The King of Personal Hygiene,* and the *OMG Teen Book Series,* starting with *OMG I'm a Teen! Now What? - A Survival Guide for Teenage Girls.*

After surviving a fatal car accident at the age of 29, Greg received what he calls "The Mission to Contribute": a calling to help others get the most out of their lives. Since then, he has dedicated his life to searching for ways to help people be the best that they can be.

Greg has over 12 years experience teaching teenagers, mostly in Thailand but also in London. One of his main areas of focus has always been to help students maximize their potential through self-assessment and goal setting.

Greg is from England, but lives a lot of the year in Thailand where he finds the beautiful beaches and mountains the perfect place for his inspirational writing.

The 5/20 Plan

Greg's major plan for the next 5 years is to inspire 20 million people around the globe to make a major change in their lives through better personal hygiene. Greg aims to achieve this goal quickly, so he can move on to helping the next 20 million people to realize their higher purpose and fulfil their greatest potential in all areas of their life.

At the forefront of this quest is educating people about the personal, financial and environmental benefits of The Bum Gun bidet sprayer.

Greg's writing focus is in the niche of Personal Development where he feels he has the biggest chance of reaching out to as many people as possible.

Cristina Noland is the Managing Director of The Fresh Wand Company, and you can find her website at www.thefreshwand.com She is an entrepreneur, housewife and keep fit lover. Huge thanks must go to Cristina for large portions of this book as it would not have been possible without her extensive knowledge of female hygiene, beauty and makeup. In fact, Cristina pressured Greg to write this book after a holiday to the UK made her realise that the local bathrooms were well behind Asia in terms of advanced hygiene facilities for females.

Cristina is passionate about raising awareness about the taboos and difficulties surrounding sanitation specifically as it relates to health and female menstrual hygiene. She is trying to stimulate dialogue about the relevance of sanitation and hygiene for female health through The Fresh Wand bidet sprayer company to break social taboos about hygiene and sanitation.

Special Bonuses

A Special Opportunity for Readers of:
"OMG – I'm A Teen! – Now What?

The OMG Teen Book Series:
I don't want our new relationship begun with this book to end suddenly. I also don't think it took you long to read this book and realize I have got a lot more information for you to learn. I could just not fit everything I have to share in this one book.

So, to keep our relationship going why don't you go on over to *The OMG Teen Book Series* website at www.omgteenbookseries.com and check on some other books in the same series. And to make the next steps even better, I would like to make you an offer.

Would you like to benefit from a 20% bonus discount from any other book in the OMG series? If so, simply email us at this email address: offers@omgteenbookseries.com to receive your voucher or look for the bonus section on our website. Simply quote voucher"**#002Teen"**

The OMG Teen Book Newsletter
Oh, by the way, it would be great if we can keep in touch. By signing up to The OMG Teen Book Newsletter at our website for the book series www.omgteenbookseries.com .We will be able to send you information on future books, free chapters, bonus vouchers and the like.

Other Books in The OMG Teen Series

Please find more information available at: OMG Teen Book Series website: www.omgteenbookseries.com

OMG My Mother! - A Relationship Guide for Teenage Girls

Greg & Cristina Noland

OMG I'm in Love! - A Dating Guide for Teenage Girls

OMG I Feel Fat! - A Health & Fitness Guide for Teenage Girls

More coming very soon…

Also, look out for 'Bertie' The Bum Gun Series (Kids)

Series 1: Bertie & Friends: The Grime Fighters

You might also like to learn more about The Bum Gun bidet sprayers at www.thebumgun.com for more information.

CPSIA information can be obtained
at www.ICGtesting.com
Printed in the USA
BVHW042109050122
625581BV00019B/440